Dedicated to "Captain Sunshine"

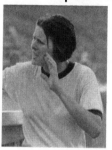

But now old friends are acting strange
They shake their heads, they say I've changed
Well something's lost, but something's gained
In living ev'ry day

Joni Mitchell
Both Sides Now, 1967

AUTHOR'S DISCLAIMER

What I have chosen to tell reflects my attempt to respect the sensibilities of those persons who, through no fault of their own, are part of my story. It is, therefore, my truth, my recollection of the events as they occurred, told to you in a good faith effort to share my experiences as I have lived them. Some names have been changed to protect the privacy of individuals.

I hope that my story will have you laughing, crying, feeling angry, feeling exalted, learning something you hadn't known and, in the end, able to include some of what I have learned in your own life.

Note:

The possessive form for many syndromes and diseases was officially eliminated in the 1980's so that Down's syndrome became Down syndrome and Huntington's disease, Huntington disease. Because many of the lay organizations were established before this was adopted, it remains possessive in the organization's official titles, and you will still see it written either way.

As a geneticist, I couldn't resist the temptation to "number" each chapter with a diagram of the corresponding chromosome number. As we humans have twenty-three pairs of chromosomes, one heads each of my twenty-two chapters. You will find the all-important sex chromosomes, X and Y, heading the Postscript and Epilogue.

While the term "mental retardation" does not sound politically correct, it is a bona fide medical designation, and is used as such.

ACKNOWLEDGMENTS

I would not have been able to tell my story without the support of my former husband. Even as he helped me with the design of this book, and grimaced at some of the more difficult memories, he generously allowed me to share details of our life together. I am grateful to my agent Rita Rosenkranz for the faith she expressed in my work, for the professionalism with which she coached me to a higher level, and for her friendship.

I owe a debt of gratitude as well to members, past and present, of my Women Who Write group. As I struggled to transition my academic voice into a personal one, their patience in reading multiple iterations was invaluable. I can still hear the late Dr. Lois Sarvetnick as she sat at the head of her dining room table insisting, "Keep going with this. You have a story worth telling." Along the way, Jana Karam stalked my passive voice, Gail Powers tracked my commas, Judy Lie asked me to define my audience, Dana Stokes found the logical order of my ideas, Mira Peck encouraged my strength as a woman scientist, and Megan Maxson lent her fresh perspective. I am grateful to Marian Calabro, author of the award-winning *Perilous Journey of the Donner Party* and founder of the custom publishing firm, Corporate History.net, for her early review and encouragement.

Neither would my story have found its proper arc without input from my sister. With her right brain's appreciation of drama, Mandy beat my left-brain into submission. I came to rely on her telling me honestly when something that I thought was clever just didn't work.

My love and forever gratitude to the many friends who lent their time to input various chapters, among them: Dawn Fontana, Michele Fabriele, Jeanne Kappel, Mary Bergen, Anne Duvoisin, Cheryl Bennett, Chuck Kaufman, Ginny Mulvihill, Sam and Joan Baily, Margery Mark, Ginny O'Donnell, Larry Golbe...

Several, including Mira Peck, Rob Palmer, and "The Boss," Roger Duvoisin, have read, and ventured feedback on the entire volume. Without "The Boss" this story would never have happened.

CONTENTS

FOREWORD
by Roger C. Duvoisin, M.D.

It is an all too human story. The initial awareness that something has gone awry is often baffling, for the diagnosis of Parkinson's disease may not become apparent for some time. In most cases, the tremor of the hand at rest with the characteristic alternating movement of thumb and fingers eventually makes the diagnosis apparent. Quite often it is the patient or a family member or friend who first notices it. Confirmation by a physician gives rise to nagging questions. Why me? How did I get it? What did I do that brought this on? What will happen to me? Can I get rid of this problem? If not, how will I live with this? Later on, more sophisticated questions arise. Did I inherit this from my parents? Have I passed this on to my children? As a scientist and student of the disease our author knew all too well the answers to these questions.

Only gradually, through a process of introspection, does one learn to accept the reality and reach a measure of accommodation and peace with the diagnosis of Parkinson's disease. As is the case with most other late-life ills of humankind, one comes to realize that it is all part of the package, an inevitable part of the human condition. It is perhaps reassuring that many others are similarly afflicted. At least one is not alone. Thankfully, for most patients, partial relief is available from modern medical treatment. There is as yet, alas, no cure. All that we have is alleviation of the symptoms for at least a period of some years and the hope that, through ongoing research, better treatments and even a cure may soon be found.

Our author is entitled to derive satisfaction from the realization that she helped bring that day closer for herself and for the thousands of others with whom she shares her journey.

♦♦♦

Among the ills that befall humankind, Parkinson's disease deserves our attention as a relatively common condition afflicting especially the middle aged and elderly, men perhaps slightly more often and more severely than women, in all walks of life, throughout the world.

Insidious in its onset, it progresses at a variable pace, so slowly in some that its inroads are barely perceptible over periods of many years, more rapidly in others, its progress as inexorable as aging. Though first formally recognized by the medical profession two centuries ago, this morbid entity has no doubt been transmitted down through the generations for countless millennia. It may even be older than the human race and indeed is not confined to humans for it has also, if rarely, been observed in elderly monkeys and baboons. It has become increasingly clear in the past decade that its origins lie, to a great degree, in our heredity, that is, in our genes, our DNA.

Our understanding of Parkinson's disease has gradually and steadily evolved since James Parkinson first identified the condition in his famous 1817 monograph *An Essay on the Shaking Palsy.* He described it as distinct from apoplexy (that is, stroke) or brain tumor or other disorders of the nervous system, a particular condition with an onset, pattern of progression, and typical combination of symptoms. He could only speculate on its possible cause. Parkinson expressed the hope that those who devoted themselves to studying the morbid anatomy of disease, those physicians whom today we know as pathologists, would devote their attention to this malady and clarify its causes. Over a century of work and controversy ultimately defined a characteristic pattern of degeneration: a distinct group of nerve cells in a brain area known as the substantia nigra, the hallmark of which is the presence of a characteristic inclusion, the Lewy body. However, the mechanism of the disease process remained obscure. At first a selective kind of aging of the nervous system was suspected. Through the first half of the 20th century the general belief was that the disease was caused by a viral infection or by cerebral arteriosclerosis. Then environmental pollutants were suspected and extensively studied.

The observation that patients sometimes had a similarly affected relative suggested a causative role for heredity more than a century ago, but this notion was overshadowed by competing theories. As in other late-adult onset familial disorders, progress was difficult, as the parents of patients, let alone their grandparents, are rarely available for examination nor are their medical records likely to be extant, even if they were affected. The author, a trained geneticist experienced in other hereditary disorders, played a crucial role in the initial efforts to clarify the genetic basis of Parkinson's disease. She worked with clinical neurologists to identify families in which cases had occurred over several generations, collected reams of information and submitted the data to genetic analysis. Then post-mortem examination documented the presence of Lewy bodies in the affected brain cells from a member of a very large family in which the disease had manifested itself in multiple individuals over several generations. The disease in this, the "Contursi family," was indeed Parkinson's disease.

The author's work with teams of scientists in the clinic and in the laboratory finally resulted in the discovery in 1997 of the first DNA mutation found to cause hereditary parkinsonism. "Teams" is the operative word, for modern genetics requires the collaborative and cumulative effort of many different disciplines over a considerable period of time. The mutation was found to be in a gene coding for an essential brain protein named *alpha-synuclein*. As one scientist put it, this discovery "blew the lid off Parkinson's research" for it opened a previously unsuspected door to the underlying biologic mechanism of the disease. And that, of course, is the *sine qua non* of ultimately finding a cure. Almost immediately brain pathologists showed that Lewy bodies consisted of a dense accumulation of *alpha-synuclein*. An astonishingly minor defect—the substitution of a single amino acid—in *alpha-synuclein* results, literally, in an improper folding of the protein that renders it resistant to the normal mechanisms for its disposal.

Misfolding of a specific protein now appears to be a feature common to several other late-life diseases of the brain like Alzheimer's and Huntington's. This has brought medical science to new therapeutic possibilities aimed at the development of drugs to prevent the accumulation of misfolded protein in the affected cells. Deciphering this mutation has made it possible to produce it in laboratory animals including mice and fruit flies. With such *transgenic* animal models scientists can study more closely the basic disease process and look for ways of preventing or correcting the defect.

XI

It was perhaps providential that the first mutation to be discovered was in the gene coding for an integral protein in Lewy body pathology. Over a dozen other mutations have since been identified in Parkinson's disease, many affecting disparate genes, and no doubt more will soon be found. Yet, the discovery of PARK1 in *alpha-synuclein* remains a beacon, the first key to unlocking the fundamental mechanism of the disease process.

One can feel in the retelling the excitement and drama of the voyage that brought us to these discoveries. Jacques Barzun referred to science as a "glorious entertainment" in his book of that title, and in some sense it truly is that. Those of us fortunate enough to have been engaged in it also know the drudgery, the hard work, the enormous time involved, and the heartbreak of failed experiments, as well as the excitement, the drama, and the glory of discovery. Add to that the wonder deriving from the special viewpoint on human existence provided by medical science and you have a heady brew indeed! Our brave pioneer enjoyed all of these and so it is all the more ironic that, at the acme of her career, she should herself become afflicted with the very same disease she had spent years studying. But this has resulted in another journey of discovery, this time, one of self-discovery.

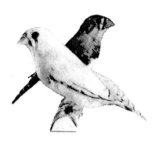

PROLOGUE
SONGBIRD

I have always been terrified of birds.

When my two children were growing up, our family took many trips into New York City where the number of pigeons exceeds the human population. It didn't take the children long to realize that they had an important role in running interference for Mommy. They'd walk ahead and chase pigeons so that I wouldn't attract undue attention by cringing and freezing in my tracks when the nearby birds began flapping their wings to fly. "Bird chasers" the children called themselves and, to this day, when they see me avoid any bird larger than a hummingbird, they chuckle and fall back into their old roles.

Fifty plus years ago, as I was growing up in West Orange, New Jersey, the town still had vestiges of its bucolic roots. Although few remain, our former neighbor's farm is still there. In the back of his tiny Cape Cod house lies a garden that once yielded such sweet carrots, even the dirt tasted good. A hand-hewn chicken coop, empty now, once housed chickens that provided the neighbors with eggs.

I must have been six or seven-years-old when the neighborhood kids chose a hot summer's day to lock me in with those chickens. I have no recollection of how they lured me there, how they got me inside or, for that matter, how I got out. I recall only the terror of being trapped in the dark sweltering heat, tiny shards of light peeking through wooden slats, and an overpowering smell of rancid hay. Indignant at my intrusion, squawking chickens flapped around my head and pecked at my feet. I wrapped my arms around my head in a vain attempt to fend off the onslaught that has left me with a lifelong fear of flying birds.

But now these winged creatures and I have a new and unexpected connection. In 1997, I was part of the Robert Wood Johnson Medical School/National Institutes of Health team that discovered the first mutation known to cause Parkinson disease in the protein known as *alpha-synuclein*. At the time of our published finding in *Science*, no one knew much about what the protein did, except as related to, of all things, the song bird. In our research paper, we wrote that, "...the equivalent protein in the zebra finch is thought to play a role in the process of song learning."

The zebra finch is part of a large family of songbirds. It is native to Australia and Indonesia, but because it breeds and does well in captivity, several research laboratories use it to investigate the neural pathways of memory and learning. As in most bird species, the male's colorful markings—his red beak and striped tail—distinguish him from the plain-looking female whom he woos with his song.

Ironically, I have now been diagnosed with the very disease I researched. Since the *alpha-synuclein* protein accumulates in Parkinson's, it is likely clogging my brain even as I write. Yet, as I journey from Parkinson's researcher to Parkinson's patient, study of this tiny bird's persistent song helps to clarify brain pathways that we have in common. One of the very creatures that have always terrified me now provides a portal through which we may learn to block and—dare we hope—reverse the process of Parkinson disease.

"Hope" is the thing with feathers
That perches in the soul -
And sings the tune without the words -
And never stops - at all —

Emily Dickinson

Chapter I
DAWNING

September 2003

The open window lets in the last breath of Indian summer as I enjoy the Sydney Opera production of *La Boheme*. From my living room armchair I imagine myself back at the Metropolitan Opera enjoying Pavarotti performing Rodolfo. My dad, an avid Pavarotti fan, had lost his mother before he was able to share the rewards of his art career with her. My son Rob had used his first earnings as a fine artist to treat his mother to the opera and I thrilled at his fulfilling his grandfather's dream.

Suddenly, my right hand begins to shake.

It stops. It starts. Stops and starts.

My hand is moving all by itself.

"Stop!"

My hand obeys.

As I melt into the music, I stop directing my hand. It begins moving again...slowly at first, then faster.

Snippets from my research career working on Parkinson disease creep into my consciousness.

A tremor in one hand that comes and goes can be an early sign of Parkinson disease.

But, how could I develop the very disease I studied?

5

Not even hearing Puccini's soaring *O Soave Fanciulla* (Oh, sweet little lady) can dispel my growing anxiety.

Shortly thereafter I go out for my early morning walk. The sun rises from behind, casting my shadow before me. I watch the shadow walking. Its left arm swings, but its right arm hangs still at its side. That can't be my shadow! My shadow has always walked with vigor. But, the next morning, my shadow does the same thing. She refuses to go away. When the sky clouds over, I watch in horror as the shadow becomes me.

Many things can cause a tremor, but a reduced arm swing is commonly the first symptom of Parkinson disease.

But that can't be. Not me!

I remind myself how medical students typically diagnose themselves with each disease they study. I must be too immersed in Parkinson's...

I had left my position at the medical school in 1999 to join the neurosciences department of a large pharmaceutical corporation. I had just begun work developing a drug for Parkinson's, and had befriended two co-workers. One was Moni Hopwood. She and I had both earned late-in-life PhDs, and we would commiserate when our more junior colleagues behaved like they didn't need our expertise. The other colleague, Enrique Carrazana, was a forty-something neurologist who mentored Moni and me. Two months earlier, Enrique had observed Moni's unbalanced gait and urged her to seek a neurological evaluation. She took his advice and consulted a prominent New York City neurologist. I was so certain that the neurologist would do some testing before making a definitive diagnosis that I did not offer to accompany her. The following morning, she told me that he had diagnosed her as having Parkinson disease after which she wandered for several hours through Central Park, alone and devastated.

The chance that two of us in a group of only thirty would develop Parkinson's within a few months' time was remote. Parkinson's starts many years before any symptoms appear. Moni and I had worked together less than two years.

I decided to tell Moni about the symptoms that I was experiencing.

"I think you've got it too," she agreed. "But, you realize, this is above and beyond the call of friendship."

Our unspoken fear of becoming dependent invalids eased by sharing, we laughed together at the huge, cruel coincidence.

"At least we're in good company with other 'Parkies' like Mohamed Ali and Pope John Paul," I told her.

Remembering the golf-cart-on-steroids that Pope John Paul used to get around, Moni offered, "We could get matching Pope-mobiles."

Then we cried together at the God-awful irony, neither of us able to give voice to a future in which we would stoop, stumble, flail, hallucinate, and perhaps become demented or psychotic.

I decided to discuss my concern with Enrique that I, too, might be developing PD.

"How old are you, Alice?" he inquired as we sat in my office, the door closed on curious co-workers.

"Sixty-three."

"Not to worry," he said, "your tremor is likely just a benign tremor of the elderly."

It was the first time the label "elderly" sounded good. I accepted his words of comfort, but knew that he was wrong. Maybe he just needed to deny the possibility that two people for whom he cared might suffer the same fate.

Later, as I walked from my office to the ladies' room, passing work cubicle after work cubicle, I noticed an odd scraping sound. I could actually *hear* a difference in the way my right foot struck the bland industrial carpet. My foot was dragging. And, it was on the same side as my tremor and reduced arm swing. I tried to ignore it but, several days later, Enrique motioned to me that he wanted to talk. He invited me into his office and shut the door.

"Alice," he asked, "have you been having any difficulty with balance?"

I had recently tripped up the stairs on at least two occasions.

"Yes," I admitted.

"Perhaps you should consider having it evaluated," he said. "I have noticed a difference in your gait."

I fought to steady my breathing as I absorbed his words. I now had three of what I knew to be the four cardinal signs of Parkinson disease: a one-sided resting tremor, slowness of movement (bradykinesia) and balance difficulties; I hadn't yet experienced the fourth, muscle rigidity, but Parkinson's was glaring me straight in the eye.

Still, I wasn't ready to seek confirmation. My son, Rob, was about to be married, and I wanted to enjoy his long-awaited special day. And, before I could even *think* about a wedding, I was expected to host an advisory board meeting during which Parkinson's specialists from throughout the world would help to plan a clinical trial for our new drug.

I had spent over 25 years in academia, written research protocols, grant applications, and papers, but had no previous experience with clinical trials. For ten of those years I coordinated a program for patients and families with Huntington disease, a neurodegenerative disorder that causes patients to writhe and flail uncontrollably. I ran support group meetings for Huntington disease families, but I had never chaired an advisory board meeting of high-powered professionals whose political agendas I didn't even want to understand. I couldn't beg off, however, lest my career come to a screeching halt.

How can I chair a meeting about Parkinson disease when I am terrified that it is happening to me?

8

I had never felt more vulnerable than when I contemplated being exposed in front of a group of physicians whose trained eyes would see my every parkinsonian movement.

Would these experts see through my charade?

Chapter II
LONDON

November 2003

I flew over the "big pond" in a luxurious, first-class seat, but was unable to sleep. After settling into my hotel room, I wanted to collapse into bed. Nevertheless, I felt compelled to find our meeting room and assure that it was set up as I had requested.

The hotel had assigned a small brightly lit room. The staff had draped the tables in white linen, arranged them in a U-shape, and set up for about thirty guests: a water glass, notepad and pen at each place, pitchers for iced-water, and little dishes of hard candy within reach. A projection screen and speaker's table stood at the front of the room facing the audience. Knowing that I would be too nervous to chair the scientific discussion and take notes at the same time, I had arranged to have the meeting recorded. The audio-visual equipment wires entwined the table legs like vines waiting to trip me.

My guests included fourteen people from my company, as well as ten from the company that co-marketed our drug, professionals from the clinical, health-regulatory, and marketing departments. Each had his or her agenda for the meeting—and for the drug. In addition, I had invited a five-member advisory board consisting of world-renowned physicians who were experts in Parkinson's. An unspoken agenda for our meeting was to get the advisory board members "pumped" about the project so as to pass on the "good news" to their colleagues, who in turn would rush to participate in our company's clinical trial.

In the weeks before the meeting, I spent hours culling the questions for our experts to address. As I prepared the slides for the two-and-a-half-day meeting, my customary stage fright kicked in. Just envisioning myself presenting the information caused my chest to tighten. I would have to get up in front of the flock of experts— neurologists who collectively had diagnosed thousands of Parkinson's patients—with my right hand shaking as it rested on the table or at my side.

Surely, I thought, *they will see it. If I am perceived as a patient and not a colleague, I will lose credibility and my hard-won career will be on the line.*

Most participants had checked into the hotel the previous day, but our department chair, Dr. Pat Sanders, was to fly in on the red-eye. She hadn't told me, but one of her confidants informed me that I was to open the meeting in her absence. Typically, performance anxiety would have kept me awake during the night. Now it was compounded with fears about holding on to my very identity as a professional.

The next morning, I showered, carefully applied my makeup, and donned my navy blue business suit, pumps and gold earrings. The hotel had set-up breakfast in our meeting room. Passing on the pastries, I poured myself coffee and took my place at the front table facing the audience. I had just begun the meeting when Pat arrived, scurrying in with her attaché and suitcase in tow and commanding attention as if she were on a red carpet. Blonde, petite, and smartly suited by Neiman Marcus, she gracefully traversed the wires that engulfed our table. A specialist in Parkinson's, she sat to my right— the side of my shaking hand.

The rest tremor of Parkinson's disappears during movement, so I knew, if need be, I could stop it by performing some purposeful action. There are, however, only so many pens to pick up, candies to reach for, or glasses of water to pour. Besides, Parkinson's specialists easily recognize these compensatory tricks. In desperation I sat on my hand when I felt it shaking. I pictured one of these doctors coming up to me during a coffee break asking:

"How long have you had that tremor?"

"Have you had any difficulty walking?"

"Have you seen a neurologist?"

Surely someone will see that I am struggling to remain the professional, but am really a patient. Could I be both? Or is my career slipping toward its own demise?

The meeting preparations, the group sensibilities, and heavily accented international discussions were the easy parts to manage. Hard was the abject fear that I might have the very disease that we were meeting to discuss. Hard was feeling as if these doctors were dissecting my brain with the casualness of their clinical discourse.

The first of our five esteemed physician-advisors began, "We need to make sure our investigators do not rely merely on a patient's report of extraneous movements." Announcing that he was demonstrating actor Michael J. Fox's dance-like movements, the physician waved his arms and made his body writhe, looking rather like a heron attempting flight.

How can he be so cavalier, impersonating a suffering patient?

Over time medications that Parkinson's patients require just to be able to move and perform the simplest of tasks become harder to adjust and they lose their effectiveness. Particularly with younger-onset patients like Fox, increasing the dose results in flailing movements called "dyskinesias."

Participants at such clinical gatherings often stoop to black humor or other such behaviors, which, in front of a patient, would violate professional standards of conduct. But, to me, his demonstration seemed mocking. I was appalled at his insensitivity. No one in the audience required his antics to understand his point. Had I remained securely in the clinical camp, I might not have reacted so critically. But, with one foot in the patient landscape, his display was too

13

graphic a reminder of what lay ahead for me.

Can this doctor even imagine what it's like to be a patient in need of medication that makes you move uncontrollably?

I had once taken comfort that there was no Huntington disease (HD) in my own family; I was not at risk to develop HD, and to flail wildly attracting gawking onlookers. HD patients endure the stares of casual observers who just assume that a wobbly gait and uncontrolled movements mean drunkenness. At least, as someone with Parkinson's, I would be rigid and draw less attention in a crowd.

But, eventually, will the Parkinson's medication that I need just to eat and dress myself make me flail and look as if I have Huntington disease?

"I'm convinced that we should measure quality of life," a second physician-advisor offered. "It is correlated with functional decline. PD patients get depressed when they go out in public and others stare at their masked faces."

How devastating would it be for my face to be so rigid that, try as I might, I wouldn't be able to smile at my family and friends? One day will I be unwilling to go out in public?

"The presence of dyskinesias is a marker of really bad things to come," pronounced Pat, not once, but frequently throughout the meeting. At least she refrained from imitation. Pat was vested in emphasizing the importance of dyskinesias as a dire entity to avoid— an entity worthy of millions of dollars for research and development, to be followed by millions of dollars for marketing.

Exactly what bad things is she talking about? How bad could they really be?

"Most of the time when we do brain surgery to ablate cells in Parkinson disease, it is because the dyskinesias are so debilitating," said the doctor who had impersonated Fox's movements, cutting deeper into my heart.

I'm not sure I can listen to this.

Referring to muscle spasms that usually occur in the extremities, another physician suggested, "Dystonias might help to get an indication from the health authorities."

That's those weird cramps I've been feeling in my legs.

As clinicians treating patients, they had to know the anguish—didn't they? I had once been on their side—the side on which it happens to someone else. Yes, you care, you feel the other's pain, you may even cry with them. Then you go home at night and you are still normal.

After two-and-a-half grueling days, the meeting was at last finished. I felt exhausted physically and drained emotionally. I longed to connect with someone who knew what I was going through. London's bleak sky and slow rain did nothing to lift my mood as I hurried to the book department at Harrods and found the last copy of Michael J. Fox's, *Lucky Man*. In it, Fox shares his ongoing battle with Parkinson's. With science showing that seventy percent of critical brain cells have died before one is even diagnosed, I needed to know how he could call that lucky.

I spent the rest of the day curled up in bed in my hotel room reading Fox's book. He talked about struggling with denial, and he captured moments for which he truly felt lucky. His irreverent reference to visiting "wizened, curmudgeonly "Dr. Big Muckety-Muck," whom I recognized as the very doctor I had just witnessed imitating him, was salve to my soul. None of us is above the vicissitudes of life—be it celebrity, researcher, or well-known doctor—and Fox obviously thought the same way.

Will I one day feel "profoundly enriched" by this "neuro-physiological catastrophe," as Fox did? Will I ever again think of myself as a lucky woman?

On the flight home from the meeting, I decided that I needed to tell my boss about my concerns. Whatever the consequences, even the end of a successful career, I could no longer maintain the deception that nothing was wrong.

Pat adopted a reassuring, if condescending, tone, "Lots of things can cause tremor. Are you sure it's not 'medical school syndrome?'"

"I have a unilateral, right-sided resting tremor, reduced right arm swing, right-sided foot drop, and some difficulty with balance," I told her in rapid-fire, to preclude her discounting my knowledge of Parkinson disease.

"I see," she replied.

I knew she knew. She knew I knew.

To break the awkward pause that followed, I asked her, "What do you think about my asking one of my former colleagues at the medical school to diagnose a friend?"

"Well, I have treated some colleagues," Pat replied with hesitation, "but it is perhaps kinder not to put your medical school colleagues in the position of having to do that." She wished me luck, then coolly turned back to the files on her desk.

Still unsure, I asked my daughter, Kathi, for her thoughts about asking a colleague to take me on as a patient. Because Kathi is both a radiologist and a psychiatrist, our family affectionately refers to her as "Doctor-Doctor." She offers a wise serenity whenever she wears one of her doctor hats with our family.

"Mom, why don't you just come out and ask your colleague if she'd be comfortable evaluating you for Parkinson disease?" Then, "You know, if you go for a diagnosis before Rob's wedding you might get treatment for the tremor and you'd feel much better."

"The tremor doesn't bother me. I'm more concerned about what lies ahead."

"If you get the tremor treated, it will take your mind off focusing on what lies ahead. And, you'll be able to enjoy the wedding," she advised.

I realized, only in hindsight, that Kathi's urging was also aimed at ruling out the possibility of something more serious than PD, something like a brain tumor. I hadn't even considered that her advice reflected a more immediate concern for my well-being. Her worry had eluded me, and I chose rather to set aside all things parkinsonian in order to enjoy my son's big step and the addition of my new daughter-in-law to our family.

That sunny wedding day in May 2004, I was gloriously preoccupied. Indeed, I forgot my concerns and relished the day's festivities.

But, my symptoms did not go away. I continued to have a tremor in my right hand, continued to observe a slowness of movement in my right arm and leg, and I had to catch my balance if I turned rapidly or bent to reach for something. I had to steel myself for the eventual reality of hearing the words, "You have Parkinson disease."

Chapter III
DIAGNOSIS

July 2004

"What the fuck does he think he's doing?" she growled. "He's a fucking asshole if he thinks I'm going to do it for him!" She stormed off the elevator fuming at her new boss and oblivious to the shock and embarrassment on the faces of those who chanced to have the experience of riding with her.

Dr. Margery Mark was renowned for cursing within earshot of patients and faculty alike, but I was fortunate to get to know the person behind all that brashness. From 1990 until 1999, she and I had adjacent offices at the medical school and spent many evenings chatting together in her office. We commiserated on the state of our department, the frustrating paucity of research coming out of the lab that she had brought to the school, and her then tumultuous love life.

Margery reminds me of my daughter. She and Kathi are close in age. Both are very bright. Margery graduated from Yale; Kathi did both her Radiology fellowship and Psychiatry residency there, but their similarities go beyond that. They are both about five feet four and physically fit, and both have unruly, shoulder-length curly hair. Both tote backpacks and wear Birkenstock sandals. Both have disdain for traditional systems, and neither has much use for what other people think about them. Both cover up any insecurity with a tough exterior. But, on the inside, each surprises like a chewy, fruit-centered candy within its hard, glossy shell. I knew that to ask Margery to diagnose a friend would be asking a lot.

"Now, what makes you think something as foolish as that?" she asked when I finally worked up the courage to phone her with my concern.

I repeated my rapid-fire mantra to hurry past my discomfort: "Unilateral right-sided resting tremor, reduced right arm swing, right-sided foot drop, and some difficulty with balance."

"Well, come on in. Let's see how good a neurologist you are," she said. "If you fail your boards, I wouldn't be surprised." Margery's one-liner conveyed both her respect for my knowledge of neurology, and her hope that I was wrong.

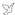

"Alice Lazzarini," Linda, the clinic coordinator announced my name to a roomful of people in the waiting area. Reluctantly standing, I felt torn between two identities. I had once called out the name of waiting patients to invite them into an examination room and toward an uncertain future. Now I was the patient and the uncertain future was mine. Old friends, Linda and I hugged, and I felt comfort behind her professional demeanor. She followed as I walked the brightly lit hallway toward where I once had counseled patients. I paused, spotting my picture on a bulletin board of photographs. Years of memories of my former research colleagues were on display for incoming patients to see. Yet, who could know the stories those pictures told?

Larry Golbe, I thought fondly, seeing pictures of the neurologist who identified the family in which we found the PD gene.

Bill Johnson. He headed the laboratory in which we began the search for the gene. He was my PhD mentor.

My God, Artiss Powell. Artiss and I had been planning to look for genes responsible for longevity, and he had just died in his 50's!

At least I'm still here.

And Dr. Tom. Tom Zimmerman and I had great fun traveling the country together to collect blood samples for research.

I miss Dr. Tom and must visit him again.

20

My trip down memory lane could postpone the inevitable only so long.

"Examination room two," Linda said, pointing to Margery's room.

I sat and waited, averting my eyes from the white-papered gurney, its wall-mounted blood pressure cuff, and blue and yellow plaid, wrap-around curtain. Closed drawers in a small table contained syringes and needles, pens, prescription pads, as well as intakes and other forms the clinician might need. How many times had I rifled these very drawers for requisite supplies?

Margery took a chart from the holder outside and entered the exam room in a single fluid motion, just as she had done a thousand times before. A barely perceptible glance of apprehension showed that this time was different. This time the chart was mine.

I stood to greet her.

"You're looking good," she offered, giving me a hug.

"And you're obviously still crewing." It was summer, and she was clad in a tight knit top and skirt above tanned, muscular legs. I remembered how her face would light up when she described six a.m. rows on Lake Carnegie in Princeton as she prepared for various crew meets.

"I'm going to need your irreverence," I told her as we sat down and she began the examination. I hoped her flippant personality could modulate the gravity of the task at hand.

"You got it," she said, her head buried in the chart as she began my intake.

"You're missing the tremor," I prompted.

"I can see it," she countered without looking up.

I handed her a family history that I had drawn on a very small piece of paper, and assured her that my family was negative for Parkinson's. "I'll leave it to you to decide whether it's micrographia"— the small handwriting, typical of Parkinson disease—"or whether I just couldn't find enough paper!" Levity, I hoped, would help relieve any discomfort either of us felt. Because she had co-authored a paper that I wrote on the genetics of Parkinson disease, she trusted my report and quickly moved on.

Wheeling her chair away from the desk, she looked at me and said, "You know the program. Here we go." Thus began the neurological examination that I had seen her perform on so many patients. "Look up. Look down. Left. Right. Well, you don't have Progressive Supranuclear Palsy," she reassured me. "Not yet."

PSP, as it is called, can look like Parkinson disease early on, but is characterized by the inability to look down. It has an even more rapid course than Parkinson's. PSP was one diagnosis I hadn't even thought of!

A litany of orders followed: "Touch my finger. Touch your nose . . . my finger . . . your nose . . . my finger . . . your nose . . . Now open and close your hand as rapidly as you can . . . Relax and let me move your arm . . . Now open and close the opposite hand . . . "

I had watched the exam so many times, I could have directed her, but I let her lead me to get the examination over with as quickly as possible.

"Now for your debut—out into the hallway. Walk down to the nurse's desk and back."

Margery invited Emily, the nurse practitioner, to join us. Emily had been waiting to see if I might qualify for entry into an NIH funded clinical trial. Income from conducting clinical trials helps to augment an academic department's bottom line, so I was not surprised by the addition of this agenda to my exam.

Soon after, Larry Golbe "happened" by. I could see by the unease in his eyes that Margery had told him I was coming and why. He, Margery and I were always close, and I knew that they would share a concern for me. Seeing sympathy in his eyes threatened to unleash emotions that I was working hard to control. I had considered asking him to diagnose me, but I could not. I would need to lean on Margery's brashness to help counter the gravity of the situation.

"I just couldn't do it to you, Lar," I blurted, as if to protect this slight, unassuming, gentle man.

22

Eight years earlier, when I was still working at the medical school, the new department chairman demanded that every faculty member bring funding into the department. I had had an NIH grant pending review, but not enough existing funding to cover my salary, so Larry shared pieces of his grants with me. His generosity extended my support for a full year before I secured a position in industry. When I left the medical school, and my new obligations made it impossible to complete a half-written paper, Larry had completed the paper and graciously credited me in the publication, noting, "The first and second authors contributed equally to this paper."[1]

Margery directed me into the hallway outside the examining room where Emily and Larry witnessed a "pull test" to assess my balance. This is typically done in the hallway where there is more room, so I had anticipated an element of being on display. However, there were no other patients at the moment, and I was among friends.

"Don't let me pull you back. Take as few steps as you can in order to keep your balance. I'll catch you if you fall," Margery instructed. She stood directly behind me and pulled my shoulders with a quick jerk. Though I had seen her do this with many patients and knew exactly what was coming, I needed three or four steps to recover my balance.

"Do it again and try to take just one step."

Again I faltered, but managed only two steps and a slight lean toward the wall. A debate ensued over whether, with questionable balance, I qualified for entry into a clinical trial designed to test two medications against a placebo or sugar pill. Balance difficulties early on increased the chance of having an atypical Parkinson's disorder. Atypical Parkinson's disorders can look like PD initially but progress more rapidly. Only their progression and autopsy differentiate them. The possibility of having something worse than PD was coming at me fast.

Heartbeat ratcheting, I asked Margery, "What are you finding?"

"I see the same thing you see: the tremor, the gait, and the arm swing," she said. "If you were a regular person, you wouldn't even be in here yet. You just know too much, that's all."

I see the same thing you see. Her understated confirmation, her clinical imprimatur, launched my new status as patient.

And yet, my breathing becoming shallower, *they are calling my questionable balance "borderline" for participation in an "early" Parkinson's trial. Might I actually have atypical Parkinson's?*

She read my concern and attempted reassurance. "The trial is set up that way because balance difficulty early on has a higher probability of being atypical Parkinson disease. But, you don't have real balance difficulty; you're just a klutz!"

I had never felt so grateful to be called a klutz. Refusing her attempt at allaying my panic was not an option. I needed to believe what she said.

The NIH-funded clinical trial for which Emily was recruiting had one last opening, and they were waiting to see if I would sign up. I was, by that time, designing and running clinical trials for industry and an avid supporter of patient participation in clinical trials.

But am I really a patient? Not yet.

Larry told me he didn't know what he would do if he were in my place. "I could envision a time down the road, if the medication proved to protect the brain, that I might regret not having taken it," he offered.

However, I reasoned, given the many PD drugs that had proven ineffective in clinical trials, it was naive to assume *this* particular drug, at *this* particular point in time, would just *happen* to be the magic bullet.

"What is involved, dose-wise if I participate in this trial?" I inquired.

"Just one pill four times a day," was Margery's answer. "No big deal."

No big deal except four times a day being reminded that I was now a patient.

I declined participation. By confirming my self-diagnosis, Margery did what I had asked. I just needed to escape, to absorb in private the impact of my transition from colleague to patient. Maybe some trial in the future would find me ready, but I was still feeling quite well. For now I wanted to focus on enjoying whatever life still had to offer.

Chapter IV
AWAKENINGS

Daybreak coaxes me awake. Once upon a time—before Parkinson's forced me to stop working—my first conscious thought was whether or not it was a workday and, if so, what I needed to do to prepare. Only on weekends could I relax, knowing that my time was my own: to food shop, straighten up the house, run to the cleaners, the bank, and perhaps the hardware store.

Now when I wake, I am acutely aware that my time is *always* my own. I can plan every day at whatever pace is comfortable—crowding in many errands or relaxing with a book. But, I realize my right arm is shaking and I am not intentionally moving it. Then a new dawning, a different kind of awakening—a realization that the movements are a time bomb that is ticking away as my brain cells die. My time is my own now *only* until that bomb goes off, until I can no longer play with my grandchildren or drive to my nephew's karate tournaments, until I can no longer move, no longer take care of myself. That is Parkinson disease. Ten, twenty, one hundred times a day when my hand begins to shake uncontrollably, that reality dawns again.

Just as in grieving the loss of a loved one, the reality of a devastating diagnosis surges in and out of consciousness in waves, as one's psyche is able to give it room. Each time the thought of Parkinson's intrudes I am surprised by its encroachment, by the absence of things as they always were. My dad has been deceased more than twenty years and my mother more than ten, yet there are still occasional moments when I am surprised to remember that they are gone. When my granddaughter is coming for a visit, for a fleeting moment I think to call Mom and invite her to join us—she loves little girls, and this charming little girl will delight her. Then I remember that Mom is no longer a phone call away.

When my mom became legally blind and could not drive, we'd grocery shop together on Saturdays. Recently at the grocery store I glimpsed an overweight, silver-haired, slightly balding woman no longer standing up to her full height. Stooping over the cookies, she appeared indecisive. Her daughter sighed, trying to hurry her decision, to get done with the shopping chore she had undertaken. Tears welled and I wanted to tell the daughter, "Please, don't rush her decision—her life—away. Someday this moment will be just a memory, and you will only see her in strangers."

When my son calls to tell me of an advance in his sculpting career, my first thought is to share it with my dad. Except for an occasional mention of "having to save pennies for drawing lessons," my dad rarely spoke about growing up an only child amidst the squalor of an impoverished neighborhood in Newark, New Jersey. I knew only that his father was a chauffeur for a family that traveled each summer from Newark to spend several months at Deal Beach. Dad's nostalgia for those summers probably explains why the only vacations we took during my childhood were day-trips to the Jersey Shore. Were Dad still

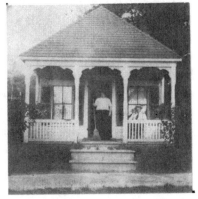

Alice & James Castles, Circa 1910

alive, I would love to ask whether our annual pause in front of a tiny whitewashed, wood-framed cottage was to acknowledge his humble origins, or whether he was picturing his beloved mother Alice sweeping the porch as his father reclined.

28

Talent and hard work had allowed Dad to leave his humble origins behind. He earned a scholarship to Parsons School of Design in New York and, after completing a three-year program in two, was invited by school founder and president Frank Alvah Parsons to join the faculty. Being offered a faculty position at one of the world's most prestigious art schools was beyond his wildest dreams. A professor first, Parsons later promoted him to Chairman of Interior Design, a career to which he devoted himself for more than forty years.

Dad commuted into New York City to teach at Parson's six days a week. On Monday through Friday he came home, changed his clothes, had dinner, and then left to teach nights at Newark School of Fine and Industrial Arts. When he returned home, he would prepare lectures and mat work for student exhibitions. As a youngster, falling off to sleep with the light from his room peeking under my bedroom door, I felt certain that I would always be safe.

I recently met a long-lost high school friend who remarked, "Your dad was a nut case!" He must have made quite an impression on her for that to be the first thing that came to her mind after fifty years. Once, my response would have been to rush to his defense. The passage of time has eased my perspective, however, and I can accept his totality. Today, a psychiatrist might diagnose him as having Obsessive Compulsive Disorder.

Forty-one when I was born, Dad was extremely protective of me. He had lived through a time when tuberculosis was a real threat and was worried that germs might harm his precious daughter. In pictures, my mom always wore white, not because she was a nurse, but because Dad had determined that white was the color of clean. Mom told me that every time I tossed a toy from my crib or play pen, he insisted she sanitize it before I could play with it again, and when she vacuumed, he demanded she send me out of the room lest I inhale germ-laden dust. When I began to walk, he allowed me only on areas of the floor covered with clean sheets. A revered colleague of my dad's once paid a visit to see his cherished offspring. The untrained visitor dared to touch me without taking off her New York, germ-tainted gloves. Despite her position of esteem, and Dad's usual obsequiousness toward people he respected, he never invited her back.

When I was a child Dad occasionally took me with him to Parsons—a forerunner of todays "bring your child to work day." My chest expanded with pride as teachers and students talked glowingly about him.

"You are Robert Castle's daughter? How lucky you are."

"Your dad is the best teacher in the school."

"How proud you must be of your dad."

"What is it like being Mr. Castle's daughter?"

And I thought to myself, if only they knew how difficult he is to live with.

Dad's over-the-top concern for my welfare and his erratic behavior caused me endless embarrassment. "If my friends see this boiling pot, I'll die," I protested, referring to the little white enamel pot he used to boil my allowance free of germs, even throughout high school. A generous weekly allowance of eight quarters dancing in that little white pot brought with it the anticipation of a fun Saturday shopping or going to the movies.

Then it happened.

My friend picked me up early. Coming in the back kitchen door, she heard my quarters clanging in the enamel pot. "What's that on the stove?" She was about to witness him drain the pot and my mortified receipt of sterilized money.

"It's my allowance being cleaned," I explained, wishing I could vanish.

"Oh," my dear friend said simply, just as she might say to this day without a hint of judgment in her voice. She didn't have to live with his idiosyncrasies!

How Dad thought he could protect me from receiving dirty

money as change when I spent my clean quarters or how he might sanitize paper currency was never clear. Didn't he know that all the sanitizing in the world could not guarantee protection from some things that life has in store? Didn't he realize that I would be the more vulnerable for having been over-protected?

Yes, my dad was a nut case, but he also modeled character traits that I continue to live by. He showed me class, humor, tenacity, taste, ambition, and integrity—and his obsessive, meticulous attention to detail would one day serve me well as a research scientist.

Before her brother became president, Kathleen Kennedy had been a student of my dad's. Dad would tell of Jack Kennedy coming to pick up his sister late one evening and waiting patiently for Kathleen to finish cleaning up her paint supplies. When they left together, the janitor was still sweeping up. "Good night, Hank," the future President of the United States addressed him by name. Dad held in high regard all that President Kennedy ultimately accomplished, but he most admired the respect that JFK had shown that evening for Hank.

Dad went on to credit Hank with a little known incident. During one of his student exhibitions, Dad needed a table to hold some artwork and he asked Hank to help devise something. Hank quickly assembled a table from available wood. According to Dad, the timeless Parson's Table, with its straight wide legs and simple design, was born that day from his need and Hank's talent.

Christmas was one time when Dad put aside his busy teaching schedule and truly enjoyed his family. Each year he unpacked the big plastic, light-up Santa face for the kitchen, the mix of antique and homemade ornaments, and the display that he had painted for the mantle: Santa and his reindeer on a blue-sky backdrop sprinkled with stars and snow. After church on Christmas morning, my younger sister, Mandy, and I would hurry home and open our presents so that we could drive through New York City to be with Mom's family on Long Island. Coming home one Christmas evening, we stopped in

Milburn in order to see the illuminated tree that towered outside the Lord & Taylor store. Disappointed to find the lights already off for the night, Dad found the electric box and threw the switch.

How could the magical glow that lit up that night, the feeling that someone would do anything for my happiness, not last forever?

Chapter V
STANDING TALL

"Alice, stand up straight. Shoulders back," my mother called to me every morning as I walked to get the bus to junior-high school and beyond. Slouching to hide my developing endowment, my adolescent body never cooperated when my mind directed it to stand erect, upright and proud. It was more than my nascent, introverted psyche could handle.

Her admonition to stand straight seems oddly haunting to me now. How would she respond to my having a disease that is characterized by stooped posture? She accepted her own losses—her sight and then her husband—with a calm grace and without complaint. But I was her baby, her first-born, and she always tried to protect me—not from germs, but from the bullies in my class, from any and every disappointment.

At seventeen years of age my mom, Amanda, enrolled as an interior design student at Parsons School of Design. She would recall how flattered she was when my dad, the auburn-haired professor, singled her out in class to give her extra help. He was twenty-nine. Dad had been married right out of high school to a woman I never knew existed until, as an inquisitive teen, I discovered his divorce papers. As Robert's interest in Amanda grew, they began seeing each other outside of school. The school banned any teacher, never mind a married one, from "fraternizing" with a student. Soon, Parsons gave him an ultimatum: give up his position, or give up his love. He did neither, but persuaded Mom to drop out of Parsons so that he could stay. His divorce took a while, so they didn't married for another seven years. I have some student work of Mom's that shows real promise, but she never developed her own artistic potential.

It was the 1940's, and Amanda felt fulfilled being Mrs. Robert Castle. With no air conditioning, Dad changed shirts three times a day. Pure cotton, the shirts were fresh-air-dried, then sprinkled with water, and placed in the refrigerator before ironing. To this day I retain a vivid image of Mom with a bandana tied around her head to prevent sweat from dripping on the clean shirts as she ironed. "Only seven minutes to iron each shirt," she proudly announced her record-setting speed. According to my calculations, Mom spent at least three hours of every week just keeping up with Dad's shirts.

Like many first-time parents, my parents determined to capture on film every breath, every blink of their new doll-like creation. Being too young to have any notion of what to do in front of a movie camera, I did what came naturally…nothing! The old 8 mm footage is filled with endless shots of me in the carriage—huge blue eyes, chubby cheeks and a finger curl atop my head that Mom set in place each morning. Dad held me and I did nothing; Mom held me and I did nothing. By all accounts, I did a lot of nothing, not even walking until I was sixteen months old.

My friend Ginny Schroll and I were only eighteen-months-old when my family moved to West Orange, New Jersey. My dad documented our growing friendship in those old movies. I starred in one neighborhood parade (after all, my father *was* the movie director) dressed smartly in my 1940's striped-bibbed-shorts and carrying an American flag. Jimmy, who lived across the street, carried his pet kitten, and Peter, from next door, lagged shyly behind. Those movies carry many memories, but so much escaped their capture.

Growing up, the neighborhood kids spent many a hot summer evening gathered "out back" behind Ginny's father's vegetable garden playing volleyball. We'd also raid the garden and enjoy the succulent taste of freshly picked vegetables. I recall, too, lazy summer days playing croquet. I can hear the "thwack" of balls being hit from hoop to hoop as we competed to be the croquet champ *du jour*. Years later, when good fortune found Mom, Mandy and me touring the Cotswold's in England, a bed-and-breakfast at which we stayed offered an unexpected croquet field. Mom, then seventy-four, was legally blind. She claimed she couldn't see a bloody cow in the road, but somehow she managed to beat Mandy and me and was the croquet champ that day. Neither Mandy nor I deliberately lost.

Mom told me that when I was a baby she secretly took me on the "germy" bus and train to visit her family in Brooklyn. She figured what Dad didn't know wouldn't hurt him—or us. That, of course, became more complicated once I began to talk. "Pop Pop gay me dis," I announced one day, blowing Mom's cover to show off a new toy Grandpa had given me. Dad was furious and told Mom not to take me to Brooklyn unless he drove us in his clean car. Nevertheless, Mom continued her clandestine defiance.

The year I was to graduate from high school Dad took students to Paris for the Parson's summer program. "Alice," he said shortly before he left, "since the car will just sit in the garage all summer long, I'm going to disconnect the battery. Hold the flashlight for me so I can see what I'm doing." While he always praised my ingenuity, he somehow didn't realize that as I held his light I was also watching how he disconnected the terminals. No sooner had he left than I was out in the garage reconnecting the battery.

Mom had recently taken driving lessons and had a license, but she was too intimidated by Dad to accumulate much experience behind the wheel. Just shy of seventeen, I had a permit and was more excited than I was nervous about driving. My high school boyfriend, Mark, also had a driving permit. While Dad was in Europe, the three of us decided to share a drive to see the college that I planned to attend in Marietta, Ohio. Eleven-year-old Mandy came along on our adventure. Each of the seven single-lane tunnels crossing Pennsylvania challenged Mom, particularly in the presence of freight trucks. She would pull off the road, Mark or I would take the wheel to drive through the tunnel, then Mom would resume the open-road driving.

Just before Dad returned from Europe I had had my first "fender bender." I scrambled to get the car repaired, and to disconnect the battery again, before his arrival. He never noticed the odometer and it was quite a few years before we told him the story of our cross-country adventure. By that time, the immediacy was lost and he let it pass. I think, too, he secretly delighted in my resourcefulness.

The gentlest of souls, Mom had to have been frustrated by the control that Dad exercised over her and over her childrearing, yet she deferred to his twelve-year seniority in their relationship. Throughout her lifetime, she retained the gratitude and deference in having won her professor and admonished Mandy and me not to express anger at Dad. Excusing his controlling behavior as overwork, she'd tell us, "Your dad teaches day and night to provide for us. You mustn't be angry at him." On occasion I begged Mom to leave him so that we might be free of his need to control. It simply was not in her repertoire to leave. She taught me this lesson well.

My dad's aunt, Alfreda had helped to secure his scholarship to Parsons. She was an independent thinking professional who had graduated teacher's college in the late 1800's back when it was known as "normal school." She became an art teacher in Newark, where she met my dad's uncle, Bob. I never saw her without a bodice laced up to her chin and wearing thick-heeled granny shoes. Perhaps she was attractive in her youth, but my memory permits only the image of a large, austere, darkly clad figure that perfectly matched the heavily draped parlor in their large Victorian home in Short Hills.

Just as Alfreda had been instrumental in launching my Dad's career, so she would influence me. "You don't want to be a *Hausfrau* like your mother!" she insisted. Those were fighting words to one who idolized her mother, but her prodding left me vowing that one day I *would* be more than Mrs. Somebody-or-other.

When Aunt Alfreda passed away my parents inherited a fruit bowl. It is the only tangible, yet oddly delicate, remembrance of an indomitable force in our lives.

I treasure the memory of Mom's good-nature, the spunk and defiance that she taught me, but how I long to hear her say, "You, Alice, YOU have the power to set your own boundaries regarding how people treat you. Your posture may become stooped, but do not let it be the fearful slouch of a victim. Be someone at peace with who you are and you'll stand tall."

Sadly, she never conveyed this message.

Now, of course, she cannot and I must tell it to myself.

Chapter VI
ON BECOMING A SCIENTIST

"I can't go to school today," Ginny said when she called. "Mom died last night." My friend Ginny and I were sixteen. Ginny's mother, Marie, was forty-five. She had had exploratory surgery for cancer the day before. There was no cancer found, but Marie died during the night as a result of the surgery. I felt utterly helpless. Helplessness changed into anger when I learned that it was ineptness that had so needlessly robbed my friend of her mother.

Ginny's mom had once run over her pet duck with a 1950 Studebaker. We joked that with her odd, backwards-looking car Marie hadn't known which way she was driving. But, Marie's death was Ginny's and my first encounter with a loss that was devastating, immobilizing. Nothing could bring her mom back, but I longed to do something, anything to ease my friend's pain. My mom taught us both how to crochet and play canasta; she sympathized with Ginny's teenage dilemmas, but my mom could not begin to replace Ginny's own mom. My effort to come to grips with Ginny's loss began a personal crusade. I vowed to take part in researching a cure for cancer.

When Ginny and I were in sixth grade, Ginny's Aunt Minnie had been assigned to substitute-teach for the greater part of our school year. She was a graduate of Mount Holyoke College, class of 1924. At a time when most women were content to be homemakers, she prided herself on being a college graduate and an activist for the

American Association of University Women. Whenever Aunt Minnie telephoned our home Mom knew that someone had likely died, as she seemed to call only when she had dire news to report. Paul Revere-like, Aunt Minnie knew it was her God-given responsibility to be the first to deliver the news.

Aunt Minnie had many quirks that gave people who knew her fodder for jest, but her prudish, matronly look belied an adventurous spirit within. Sixth-grade boys lie in wait to take advantage of any teacher that betrays the slightest vulnerability, so Aunt Minnie became the butt of many pranks. I remember the day my classmates tested her limits by hiding a can of live, crawling worms in her desk, and then sat in gleeful anticipation of her gasp of revulsion. To their dismay, Aunt Minnie took the unexpected opportunity to teach the class about how worms eat and recycle the dirt around them. She was a true field biologist. As much as we joked at her expense, I completed that sixth grade year with a genuine enthusiasm for biology. To this day I credit Aunt Minnie's field trip to collect tadpoles from a local pond, and the exhilaration of watching those tadpoles magically transform into frogs, as the seed from which my love of science germinated.

Ms. Gardner, my freshman biology teacher, was another kernel in my scientific development. Well, maybe not exactly Ms. Gardner. She had a student teacher with her that year: Mr. Napoli. Somewhat stocky, bespectacled, probably all of twenty years of age, Mr. Napoli was the most beautiful thing my teen-age self could imagine. He showed me the organized way in which all plants and animals fit together in a grand universal plan. He escorted us on wonderful field trips. I still have pictures taken with my Instamatic camera—images frozen in time, as if to deny that he is likely now an overweight aging grandfather.

In my junior year in high school, I had another beautiful, young male teacher for inorganic chemistry. Mr. Worthington showed me the periodic table, a system in which each element occupied its own place in a perfectly ordered world, and I blossomed under his tutelage.

Two other high-school friends lost their mothers to colon cancer, and then the unthinkable happened. One of our peers developed bone cancer and had a leg amputated. Graduation found him struggling to the stage on crutches to receive his diploma amidst stirring applause. Just as with Ginny's mother, my sadness over his plight fed my resolve to contribute to cancer research. There was no doubt that I would attend college and major in science.

I began my college career by heading west to Marietta College in Ohio. The freshman class in my major, chemistry, was in a lecture hall of some 120 students. Beyond the rows of students, I could barely see the stodgy, uninspiring professor. I felt lost. The other students seemed more adept at assimilating this new subject material than I. More homesick than I could have imagined, I begged my parents to let me come home after six months. In conjunction with the school counselors, they insisted that I give it a full year. At the end of the year I came home with my "C" in chemistry, and a desperate need to overcome feelings of failure.

Trying to regroup, I attended a local junior college where I met Marsha Myers, a kind, nurturing biology teacher. This time the object of my feminine urges was a fellow student, a tall Irishman named Danny, who had attended Annapolis. He showed me his class photo, looking beautiful in his uniform, and I was smitten. He was four years my senior. Together we were taking Dr. Myer's Comparative Anatomy course in which we got to share the dissection of a two-foot long dogfish shark. We named our shark "Charlie." One evening, I suggested that we work on dissecting Charlie at my parents' house. Mom agreed, but then Dad came home. The pungent odor of formaldehyde led him straight to us. Seeing Charlie splayed in an aluminum pan, only a thin pad protecting his precious cherry dining room table, he demanded, "Get that God-awful smelly thing out of here." Marsha, Danny, and the wonders of Charlie's intricate anatomy, helped me to realize that studying biology was the perfect choice for me. By triggering defiance, my father only fed a determination to forge my own path.

41

Marsha steered me toward the biology program at the College of St. Elizabeth where she had once taught. There I met Sister Anna Catherine. Sister was a formidable figure, her face squarely cornered by the rigidly fluted wimple that was still worn by the Sisters of Charity in the early sixties. We fondly called her "Anna Cat," although never directly to her face. When Anna Cat had neck surgery one year, she insisted on being awake throughout so that she could watch and, we students were sure, direct the procedure. She insisted "her girls" toe the mark and, after long days in class, many an evening was spent finishing up one or another of our laboratory experiments. She made sure we were aware that she had earned a PhD from Columbia, having studied with Theodore Dobshansky, the geneticist who authored one of our textbooks. I thrived on Anna Cat's encouragement, and the hard work she demanded felt like a perfect fit.

In my senior year Anna Cat made a request for someone to provide a cat with which we might study histology. Histology is the study of cells and tissues, which meant, of course, sacrificing a furry feline. Laboratory cats that were already preserved were provided for some studies, but for histology the tissues had to be fresh and each one stained with its own specific dye. The dyes help to visualize each beautifully ordered structure under the microscope. I was so swept up by the prospect of being witness to the inner workings of an animal as large as a cat that I put aside my compassion for all small creatures, as well as any intimidation at approaching a very eccentric neighbor for help.

Miss Kimball lived in a weathered Victorian house with only her pet cats for company. She must have been in her late seventies, but did not allow her age—or diminutive height—to deter her from driving. She drove a huge green 1953 Buick Roadmaster very slowly around the neighborhood—probably only to church and back. However, Miss Kimball was so short you could not see her behind the wheel! Seeing that car with the silver, gill-like side vents bearing down the street with no driver, I reasoned that if I couldn't see her inside the car she likely wasn't able to see much outside the car.

Miss Kimball's annual moment of fame came at the St. Cloud Presbyterian Church Festival. Replete with turban, tattered gypsy-like clothes, a large "crystal" ball, and some smoking dry ice she was the fortuneteller. Her raspy voice lent just the right aura as she hawked, "Come here little one. Let me tell your fortune today." Half the fun for the neighborhood kids was daring each other to approach her. Maybe she really did have magical powers. I never mustered the courage to go anywhere near that table.

When she was not driving or telling fortunes, Miss Kimball tended to her cats, probably twenty or thirty of them. If Anna Cat needed a cat for our course in histology, it seemed quite logical to me to ask Miss Kimball to donate one. After all, she had plenty to spare. Besides, I could earn brownie points if I provided a cat for the entire class. This time, my enthusiasm outweighed my timidity, and I worked up my courage to approach Miss Kimball. I sauntered through the woods that separated our properties, and I invited her to make a contribution to my cause.

"You want to kill one of my cats?" her raspy voice screamed. I was sure the entire neighborhood heard my mortifying rejection.

Mumbling an embarrassed, "I'm sorry," I crept back home through the woods.

Someone else donated a cat for histology, and I persisted in my studies undeterred. Constantly sharpened pastel pencils meticulously rendered the details of each tissue structure, many of which I can picture to this day.

Long before human genes were introduced into animals and models constructed to facilitate the understanding of human diseases, Sister Anna Catherine taught us to conduct cancer research experiments in mice. By injecting tissue that had been filtered, we showed that particles as small as viruses could transmit cancer from mouse to mouse. I felt sure that the brass ring of understanding how cancer might be caused, and possibly cured, was there for the grasping.

In our genetics course I learned how to culture fruit flies, mate them, and record changes in the offspring. Because of their short life span and ease of manipulation, their study is a very important tool for geneticists. The feelings of ineptness that I had carried from Marietta College receded, as I became adept at performing these experiments.

On February 20, 1962, I arose early. Anna Cat was driving a group of her girls to Syracuse University. We were scheduled to present our research results at a conference of Beta Beta Beta, a national biology honor society.

John Glenn had arisen even earlier. It was the day he took the first orbital flight aboard Friendship 7. En route to Syracuse, we all held our breath as we listened to the live broadcast of the launch. The nation had heard continual coverage leading up to the historic event. Would Glenn be able to go out beyond our atmosphere and return safely? I was nervous for him and nervous for me. I had never before presented a paper.

After several suspenseful hours of mission delays the voice of NASA's Mercury Control crackled over Sister's car radio, "Glenn reports all spacecraft systems go. Mercury Control is go!"

"The view is tremendous," we heard Glenn exclaim.

I, too, had a newfound view of the world. I was now a scientist who had something to contribute that others would gather to hear. I felt sure my exhilaration that day matched John Glenn's own.

Chapter VII
HE'LL ALWAYS TAKE CARE OF YOU

September 1962...

Sister Anna Catherine had personally steered each one of her girls toward the careers that she envisioned for them. She had hand picked those she saw as physicians and those that she saw pursuing research. I fit into the latter category and was awarded a graduate fellowship at St. John's University on Long Island. St. John's turned out to be a re-enactment of the failure that I had experienced at Marietta. However, it was at St. John's that I met the man who would become my husband.

To earn a PhD in biology, I was required to take a course in physiology for which an undergraduate course in physics was a prerequisite. But I had not had physics as an undergraduate. "Physics is not for girls," I distinctly remember Sister Anna Cat telling me. Only in retrospect did I question the idea that, in order to earn a PhD in genetics from Columbia, she had to have taken physics and, underneath that wimple, I felt certain that she was a girl. I had no choice but to enroll for graduate physiology and undergraduate physics concurrently.

In my physics class there was a handsome young fellow whose name was Bob, just like my dad. A second-generation Italian, he was olive-skinned and sported large, dark-rimmed glasses. He worked part time supplying equipment for the biology department's laboratories. Sitting next to him class, I remember being distracted from the lecture by the little hairs on the back of his hand. He was still an undergraduate, but he was very attentive, making a point of talking to me after every class. There were several other good-looking guys in the graduate program—big shots just like me. However, there was something charming and endearing about this cute, bespectacled undergraduate with his crisp, white lab coat flying as he marched purposefully down the halls.

As a woman in the 1960's and in science, I was feeling pretty special. Coming from the shelter of a private Catholic girl's college and living on my own in the Big Apple (albeit Queens, Long Island), I was heady with my newfound status as a graduate student receiving a stipend for teaching lowly undergrads.

"I really don't get that last physics lecture," I told Bob one evening after class.

"I can help you with it," he replied.

"That'd be great," I told him. Soon I was driving to his house for regular study sessions. He commuted the ten miles to school by bus, but I had my own car—a '57 Ford Fairlane.

Bob's mom, Helen, barely five feet tall with dyed black hair, spoke loudly and imposed her opinions with a righteousness that precluded debate. She ruled with an iron fist, literally punching her two sons into submission, berating her meek, first-generation immigrant husband, and generally creating chaos from calm. Her roost had plastic covers on the furniture, blinds on the windows, and wall-to-wall carpeting. I had come from a home in which sheets protecting furniture were removed when company came, shades graced the windows, area rugs revealed oak floors, and anger was repressed.

Helen couldn't believe her good fortune that her son had found a bright, ambitious, clean-cut girl, and she welcomed us sitting around her kitchen table for endless study sessions. Each session ended with her offering delicious lasagna, Chicken Parmesan, or Veal Marsala. Despite my grownup independence, my car, my apartment, and my graduate status, there was comfort in that home cooking. For many years, I did not see past the comfort to what lay beneath. Neither did

46

I foresee the degree to which human behavior can be passed from generation to generation.

Bob's interest was more than physics, more than comfort. He says to this day that he just knew that I was the one for him. He was twenty. I was twenty-one. Until that time, I had had two serious relationships. The last, and most devastating, had ended with a "Dear Alice" long-distance phone call on my twenty-first birthday. I was left hurt, confused, and needing consolation.

While Bob needed his mother's approval, he also needed to get out from under her control. I was unaware at the time, but he was also struggling to keep up with several of his courses at St. John's. His mother had refused to pay for his college unless he took pre-med. His dad was unable to provide guidance, but simply deferred to Helen on all matters "American." One solution would have been for Bob to strike out on his own by getting a job and going to school at night. He wanted to study art, but Helen grasped at the interest he had expressed in science to steer him toward the goal of having her son become a physician. He would have made a wonderful naturalist—a photographer for National Geographic, perhaps. Instead, I was his out.

Upon starting graduate school, I had found an apartment in a private home. I had no sooner moved in than I awoke one morning with the landlady's adult son standing over me. He just stood there, staring down at me. My screams sent him scurrying for the door, but I was left unnerved. He had somehow gotten his mother's key and decided to let himself in. My landlady apologized and refunded my money, but I had to find another apartment, just as my grueling class schedule had begun. Mom came in from New Jersey and my dear Aunt Ellie came from Brooklyn. Together they helped me to find a new apartment and move in. After an entire day of their cleaning and setting up, Dad came to see my new apartment. To his chagrin he discovered that it overlooked a former tuberculosis hospital. "You can't stay here. You'll catch TB," he declared, even though the hospital had not treated tuberculosis in years.

It was easier to do what he demanded. God knows why—habit, I guess. We acquiesced and found an apartment on the opposite side of the same building. Somehow that distance satisfied his irrational concern. So Mom, Auntie, and Bob packed up my belongings and hauled everything from one end of the building to the other.

"Here, Mrs. Castle, let me carry that heavy box for you," Bob said, taking a carton from her. He was trying hard to impress the women whom he aspired to calling 'Mom' and 'Auntie,' but he had failed to support the box bottom. The cacophony of pots and pans hitting the floor did anything but impress.

"He's very young," was all that Mom said when he was out of earshot. She was to repeat the same astute observation many times over the years. We were both young. Our needs—his for escape and approval, mine for love and devotion—were strong and we soon became romantically involved.

"I'll have a Jack Daniels," I told him one evening when we were out bowling with his friends. I was a graduate student out to show off my sophistication to these mere undergrads. Bob had expected me to ask for a coke, yet perhaps guessed from my posturing that he was involved with someone who wanted to be seen as strong and self-determined. However, between the stressful incident with my landlady's son, having to move three times, and not having taken physics before attempting physiology, I soon became overwhelmed. Bob did his best to tutor me in physics, but I was struggling to keep up with the complicated concepts in physiology without understanding physics. At the end of the first semester, I was "invited" to drop out of school, re-group and reapply. To me that was tantamount to another failure. I had been awarded a graduate fellowship as testimony to others' faith in me and I had blown it big time. I had let down my parents—and myself. Once again, devastation, embarrassment, and feelings of inadequacy pervaded my soul. I had trouble eating, and I lost weight.

Bob was there to love and comfort me when the boom fell. Gone was the sophisticated, independent big shot. In her stead was a vulnerable, hurting twenty-two year old little girl depending on her twenty-one year-old lover. I took my needs and joined them with Bob's. Together we made a needy couple.

When I left St. John's, I found a job working as a laboratory technician at Sloan-Kettering Institute for Cancer Research in Rye, New York. I licked my wounds, but at least I was back on track and able to see myself as a participant in science's march forward. My boss, Dr. Morris Teller, was a well-known researcher in erythropoietin, a protein that came to figure significantly in cancer treatment as well as in much of the funding for Sloan-Kettering. Erythropoietin has recently been recognized as a protective agent in brain tissue, but this was not known in 1963, nor could I have guessed what that might imply for my own future health.

Soon after I took the job in Rye, I began to find myself arriving in the morning and running to the ladies room overcome with nausea. I had missed my period and wondered if I could be pregnant. Bob and I had been together for only a few months. My mom didn't have me until after one miscarriage and five years of trying to conceive. My birth was followed by another miscarriage, and it was six years before my sister and only sibling was born. Even as a youngster I had adored little children and wanted to have my own someday. From the time I first grasped a vague concept of genetics, I had worried about having the same difficulty bearing children as my mother.

Me a mom! I began to fantasize about our little family: Bob would find a job and provide for us both. My dream of a scientific career seemed to have been derailed, but it was being replaced by another one of my dreams. And, then we had to tell my family.

Struggling to put a positive spin on the situation, Dad assured me, "He'll always take care of you," and he then went to his room to cry out his tears of disappointment in private. Dad's ambition for me was that I finish my education, make a contribution to science, and marry a professional who would provide bountifully for his firstborn. I had just demolished his dream.

"He's so young," Mom remarked again, guarding her justifiable concern. At twenty-one, Bob could still pass for a high-school student. Bob got his first job as a lab technician at Ciba Pharmaceuticals and, because he hadn't yet gotten his New Jersey driver's license, I drove him back and forth to work.

We moved our sofa bed into my parents' dining room while we readied an apartment that we had found nearby. About one week before my due date, my water broke while sitting on Mom's sofa, and Bob called her home from her part-time job in retail to drive us to the hospital.

"Can't you drive faster?" I urged.

"Not in this downpour," she cautioned. "You've got plenty of time with the first one."

Kathleen was born soon after midnight on November 8th, 1963 and I took her home for my birthday on the twelfth. She was my birthday present from God, and far and away the best present I have ever received. I did not see the compressed skull or the forceps-mark on her cheek that is present in her newborn photograph. She was the most beautiful baby I had ever seen, and grew into the most beautiful little girl. Tiny and affable, she enchanted everyone with whom she came in contact. When strangers stopped me to admire her big blue eyes and proclaim her a Gerber baby look-a-like, I opened my own blue eyes wider and puffed up with pride.

Several women whom I know have endured post-partum depression after having had glorious pregnancies. My experience was exactly the opposite. Hormonally challenged, I was irritable during my pregnancy, but once Kathi was born I soared heavenward, my heart filled with a love I cold never have imagined myself capable of feeling. I was the luckiest person alive.

Just fourteen months after Kathi was born I conceived again. My mom called Bob home from night school when I went into labor. He said that he ran every red light en route to the hospital. He held me close with each ripping pain and glowed with pride when I delivered our son. We had little money, yet he brought to me a dozen long-stem roses in a milky white vase, a testament to the pride he felt.

50

Surely he would feel fulfilled now that he had a son and namesake: Bobby.

While our pregnancies had not exactly been planned, I knew I wanted children and was thrilled being a mother. I never questioned whether Bob was ready, but assumed that if he agreed—and cooperated—he'd always take care of me, just as my dad had promised.

Chapter VIII
BECOMING A PROFESSIONAL

Back in the Sixties day-care centers were not commonplace like they are today, so I took my then five- and three-year-olds with me to volunteer at the Easter Seals Center preschool program in Morris Plains. I fell in love with little Paul, a one-year-old with Down syndrome. His mom Jackie bore a heart that was laden with worry for Paul, as well as for herself. I learned later that, in addition to a special-needs son, Jackie had a mother with late-stage Huntington disease (HD).

HD is typically a twenty-year deterioration of mind and body, characterized by loss of physical, cognitive, and emotional control. As neurological diseases go, it is one of the nastiest. Besides flailing uncontrollably, patients lose their ability to think and reason, and eventually enter a vegetative state. HD strips a person of all dignity and, because it is genetic, it reappears generation after generation. Jackie lived with a 50% risk, not only of succumbing to her mother's fate, but also of one day becoming too ill to provide for her son. And yet she remained upbeat. I came to particularly admire Jackie's positive outlook on life, and I nicknamed her "Captain Sunshine" after Neil Diamond's 1970s song.

Over the next few years, Jackie invited me to come with her to support group meetings of the Committee to Combat Huntington's Disease (CCHD).[1] At one of those meetings in the early '70s, I met Marjorie Guthrie, the widow of folk singer Woody Guthrie. Woody was probably the most well-known person to have had HD. "My dear, you must help us spread the word about this dreadful disease," Marjorie addressed me as if we were old friends.

Marjorie was a gatherer of apostles. As she spoke of once having been a Martha Graham dancer, I struggled to reconcile the image of this gracious, lady-like persona married to a folksy, guitar-slinging, train-hopping, Dust Bowl troubadour. She was the second of Guthrie's three wives and, despite their dissimilar life-styles, they maintained a close relationship until he died.

Listening to the gospel according to Marjorie, I was charmed by this woman's ability to turn personal tragedy into a cause that was to help so many. Woody had been repeatedly misdiagnosed and then suffered a humiliating decline in a series of psychiatric hospitals with little or no available resources. Marjorie meant to change all that. After Woody's death in 1967, Marjorie founded CCHD, which was the forerunner of the current Huntington's Disease Society of America (HDSA). HDSA continues to fund important research and serves as a resource from which family members can find information and support.

In 1974, Jackie and I attended a support group meeting at which we met a woman who had just completed the fledgling Genetic Counseling Program at Rutgers University. I was not even aware that such a training program existed, and I asked her to tell me about it.

"Genetic counselors learn to work with people from families in which a genetic disorder has been found or suspected," she told me. "They help family members to understand the disease, as well as its risk of recurrence, and to identify appropriate resources."

As an undergraduate majoring in biology, I had always loved genetics, fruit flies and all. To study genetics and to be able to help people in the context of a clinical setting sounded like the perfect career path for me. And Rutgers University was less than an hour's drive from my home!

Just as I had done when I left St. John's and had Kathi, I reverted to an alternate dream, this time back to my dream of a scientific career. But now it would be harder. I was also a mother and caring for two children who were then eleven and nine years old. I enrolled in the two-year Genetic Counseling Program at Rutgers.

At a subsequent CCHD meeting I met my first patient with Huntington disease. Betty had chorea (from the Greek word, to dance), the movements of HD that caused her to writhe uncontrollably throughout the entire meeting. She sat right up front and didn't seem to mind attracting attention. I introduced myself to her and was in awe of her positive attitude. My fellow graduate students were going to have to meet this lady. I invited her to participate in our program's grand rounds, an educational forum for medical professionals in training, during which patients and family members share their experiences in dealing with a given disease.

As we began grand rounds, Betty's husband, John, wheeled her to the front of the lecture room. A respectful hush fell, the students unsure what to expect. Despite being beset by flailing movements, Betty answered questions freely and maintained a cheerfulness that belied her plight. "I don't mind these movements much," she told us. "They are a big help when I beat batter for a cake. Of course John has to pour it into the pans, or else I'd have a lapful."

I was charmed by her good humor, as were my fellow students. Like Jackie, she remained optimistic in the face of devastation. How could Jackie and Betty be dealt such cruel hands and remain so upbeat? I marveled at their inner strength.

After we finished grand rounds and the lecture hall had emptied, Betty asked, "I want to write a letter to the HD Commission. Could you help me?" She wanted me to help her compose a letter to the Federal Huntington's Disease Commission, a needs-assessment agency that had been set up in 1972 in order to determine how federal monies might best be used to meet the needs of HD patients and their families.

One blustery fall day, I brought my son with me to Betty's home. John sat on the floor with young Bobby and delighted him with his World War II plane models. Betty and I composed a letter elucidating her plight, and that of other HD families, in which we emphasized the desperate need for research funding in order to find a cure. Being with Betty and John felt cozy, comfortable and oh so right. This was the beginning of my long involvement with a much larger HD family. Betty's plight was my plight; we had to find a cure. Admiration had made me a committed advocate, and throughout my genetic counseling training I would retain a focused interest in working with HD.

In 1974 Michael K. McCormack, who had just received a PhD from the University of Minnesota, came back to his home state of New Jersey to join the faculty of the Genetic Counseling Program at Rutgers University. The timing of Mike's return to New Jersey was perfect, and his influence on me, profound. He became my teacher and first mentor.

Sheldon Reed, Mike's mentor at Minnesota, had coined the phrase "genetic counseling" and was defining this burgeoning new field. I could not have had a more direct line of descent in my proposed field—a direct connection to the man who became known as the "Father of Genetic Counseling." Reed's mentor in turn was William E. Castle, an early twentieth-century geneticist who was the first to use the fruit fly as a genetics tool. Castle had founded the journal *Genetics* and published the last of his 242 papers when he was ninety-one years of age. My maiden name was Castle. While I never found a connection between my family and William Castle's, at least my professional pedigree related back to the head honcho.

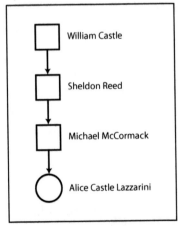

My professional pedigree

I would later introduce genetics lectures using a diagram of my professional pedigree emphasizing the gender change—from a square (male) to a circle (female)—at the end. I thrilled with the certainty that my career choice was somehow predestined.

By 1975 Mike and his fellow University of Minnesota graduate student, Ann Willey, together with clinician Ming Liang Lee and cytogeneticist, Leonard Sciorra, had parlayed the genetic counseling training program at Rutgers University into a clinical service within the Department of Pediatrics at what was then Rutgers Medical School.[2] Together they covered the key disciplines within genetics: clinical, biochemical, and cyto (or cellular) genetics. Within medicine, genetics is unique in that it requires an enormous amount of time spent with the patient. One frequently needs to treat—or at least take into account—an entire family. Even before the days of managed care, getting reimbursement from insurance companies to cover the cost of time spent counseling a patient was a pressing issue.

Lenny and Ann are both cytogeneticists and study chromosomes, the structures that contain our genes. Together they set up a laboratory devoted to culturing cells and affixing chromosomes from those cells onto glass slides in order to view and photograph them under a microscope. The cells might be from babies with suspected syndromes such as Down syndrome, in which there was an extra chromosome number 21. Alternatively, the cells could be from people with certain cancers, or amniocentesis samples from women of advanced maternal age, "AMA" as we glibly referred to it. Studies had determined that thirty-five was the age at which a woman's risk of having a baby with Down syndrome exceeded her risk for the amniocentesis procedure. AMA for prenatal chromosome testing constituted a frequent referral for genetic counseling.

When chromosome preparations are made, the cells are dropped onto a microscope slide. When viewed under a microscope, the 46 chromosomes within each cell have literally fallen every which way. Clear, relatively non-overlapping chromosome spreads are what a laboratory technologist hopes to find in his or her laborious, grid-by-grid search of the slide.

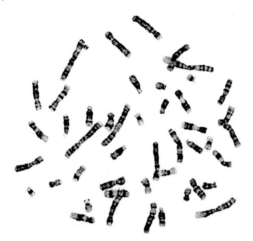

Chromosome spread as viewed under a microscope

In order to properly assess their content, the 46 chromosomes from a single cell are then grouped from largest to smallest, arranged in pairs into a "karyotype," and their content interpreted. Any medical consequences of similar known abnormalities can then be referenced in discussing findings with the family. These procedures—as opposed to time spent just "talking"—were recognized and reimbursed by insurance companies. In those early days, the cytogenetics laboratory carried much of the weight of funding for the entire clinical genetics program.

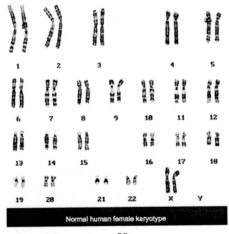

Normal human female karyotype

Ann Willey is a tiny, unassuming powerhouse, her fine, blond hair hanging straight around a pale face, obscured by large, slightly outdated glasses. Perhaps the most laid back person I have known, she often looks as if she had thrown on whatever outfit her hand happened to land on when she reached into her closet that morning. But, her warmth makes you feel like the only person who matters. When she speaks, you know that you are in the presence of a genius—a caring and generous genius.

Lenny sports a scruffy salt-and-pepper beard on a face scarred from teenage acne. Underneath a mane of straggly hair and tousled attire, this brilliant scientist delights in being able to pass for the janitor or handyman. Lenny rose from humble beginnings to receive his PhD from Hahnemann University in Philadelphia. In 1976, when the movie Rocky came out, he identified with Sylvester Stallone's downtrodden hero Rocky Balboa, and the soundtrack of Stallone's triumphant run up the steps of the Philadelphia Museum of Art was played incessantly in Lenny's laboratory. "Yo, Adrian" became his too-often quoted favorite line.

One day I accidentally intruded upon Ann and Lenny huddled in the small darkroom that he had set up. She had been crying. "Mike just told me that this program can support only one cytogeneticist," she sobbed. "He's able to keep only Lenny."

Now you may question her crying on the shoulder of a competitor, but Lenny is a gentle soul who, were the decision left to him, would likely have found some way to support them both. I was devastated for my friend, Ann. And, I was shocked that Mike, Lenny and Ann's Three-Musketeer-like group could be so easily dismantled. After recovering from her trauma, Ann went on to direct New York State's proficiency program in cytogenetics. Every laboratory that received clinical samples from patients living in New York—and that included Lenny's—must adhere to and pass her proficiency exams. When little Annie did her spot checks, many a mighty lab head would quake in fear. Not content with one high-powered position however, she also went on to study and then teach law. She has remained a dear friend.

Bob had encouraged me to return to school, and he pitched in, being present for the kids after school or on evenings when I had to study or complete a school project. Upon finishing my master's, I determined to once again begin working on my PhD. However, I no sooner registered and began classes when Bob came home with news that he had been fired. Once again my aspiration to complete a PhD was thwarted. Would I ever finish my doctorate, or was fate conspiring against me? Rather than continuing my life as a student, I was faced with the need to find a salaried job in order to cover our household expenses.

I turned to Lenny with my plight, and he provided me with a position in his cytogenetics laboratory. After culturing cells and preparing chromosomes, I photographed them under the microscope, developed the film, and printed the pictures. Ever the ingenious handyman, Lenny had converted a bathroom in our building into a darkroom for developing the chromosome photographs. Because film developing is temperature sensitive, he warned, "You'll just have to remember to adjust for changes in water temperature if you hear someone flushing the toilet on the floor above you."

Lenny gave me great flexibility in deciding when I was able to get the work done. During the summers when Kathi and Rob were off from school, I left home at 4 am and drove an hour to the lab in the dark. To this day the sound of birds chirping before sunrise transports me back to those early morning drives to the cytogenetics laboratory. I would work as quickly as I could, then head home in time to pick up the children when their summer music program ended at noon.

My briefcase, reeking of fixative, was stuffed with newly developed pictures of chromosome spreads to cut out and arrange into karyotypes. Today karyotyping of chromosomes is done on the computer, but back in the seventies computer manipulation of chromosomes was not yet perfected. After the images were photographed and the film developed and printed, the chromosomes had to be cut out and arranged by hand. Recognizing the specific pattern that characterized each chromosome was where my training came in. Cutting them out was grunt work.

I had two kids. Two kids could be paid to cut out chromosomes. Mixing the chromosomes of different people could result in dire errors, however, so I sat Kathi in one room and Rob in another, each with a pair of scissors and the promise of a dime for each karyotype that they cut. Their doing the cutting probably saved me ten minutes on each one; all that I had to do then was to arrange and tape the chromosomes onto the template. At the time, I probably was making $10 per hour, and cleared about $9 after I paid my child laborers.

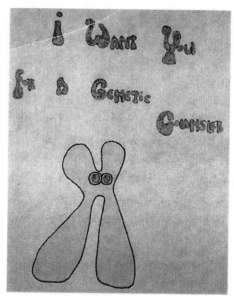

Rob's Poster, circa 1976

Kathi's familiarity with cytogenetics held her in good stead for many a summer job. When I completed my MS in Genetic Counseling, ten-year-old Rob drew me a poster with an oversized caricature of a chromosome proclaiming, "I want you for a genetic counselor." It has always commanded a special place in my office.

When she took her new position with the New York State laboratories, Ann Willey and her husband Jack bought a big, old farmhouse twenty minutes outside of Albany. It was a house that accommodated many guests—with lots of rooms and a relaxed atmosphere. In 1978, a genetics meeting held in Albany was the perfect excuse to see my dear friend again. Several former genetic-counseling students and I piled into my car and made the four-hour drive from New Jersey. Sprung loose from our everyday obligations, we sang and laughed through the entire trip. When we arrived at Ann's and Jack's, where we were to spend the night, my passengers retrieved their suitcases and headed inside. I was preparing to do the same, when I realized that a rooster was standing right outside my car door. He stared at me, paced back and forth a bit, and waited for me to get out. He was large and appeared quite sure that he belonged there, but I did not. Frozen, I could not open the door.

By now everyone was inside and, presumably, happily chatting and catching up on all the news. I sat there staring at this large, mean looking bird, thinking that even if I honked my horn, no one would hear it. How long would it be before they realized that I was missing? I was fully prepared to recline the seat and spend the night in the car.

Finally, Ann came out and shooed the rooster, laughing, "That rooster is nasty. He'll as soon take a nip at you as anything," she said. "Just steer clear of him and you'll be fine."

Steer clear I did. With every trip to and from my car, I recruited someone to be my bird chaser. "Helen, come with me to get my map from the back seat of the car," I asked.

"You really are a chicken—pun intended," Helen quipped amidst the group's teasing laughter.

🕊

When I next saw her, Ann gave me a little ceramic rooster as a memento of the occasion. Sitting on my kitchen windowsill, it reminds me of her gentle humor. It reminds me, too, of my own vulnerability.

Chapter IX
GENETIC COUNSELING

By the time of the Albany meeting, I no longer was doing strictly cytogenetic laboratory work, but also was seeing patients for genetic counseling. Many cases were for routine prenatal testing in order to rule out certain known abnormalities. Because our training had emphasized not slipping into what seemed like a canned talk, I worked at engaging each couple in the counseling process. I began by asking about their background in biology and, hence, their likely comfort level with the genetics terminology that I was about to discuss. Using diagrams and pictures, I then walked them through the rationale for doing amniocentesis, as well as what to expect during the procedure itself.

Amniocentesis usually is done between twelve and sixteen weeks of pregnancy and, once advanced maternal age (AMA) was established in the professional literature, a referral for genetic counseling became the standard of care. Obstetricians wanted to avoid being sued should a pregnancy result in a child with preventable birth defects. Couples often had been referred to us so matter-of-factly that they came in without a clear understanding of why they were even there. After counseling, an occasional mother declined prenatal testing on religious grounds, but most complied with their doctor's recommendation. Whenever I attended an amniocentesis procedure, I found myself glad that I had had my children before I was thirty-five when my age would have been advanced enough to indicate that a long needle be stuck in my belly in order to obtain amniotic fluid for testing.

With more women giving birth at a later age, the procedure itself became more routine, hence safer. By the 1980s, chorionic villus sampling (CVS) became an alternate to amniocentesis for mothers who were referred early enough. Whereas amniocentesis must wait until there is sufficient amniotic fluid around the developing fetus, CVS obtains placental cell samples through the cervix, and is done between eight and twelve weeks of pregnancy. With CVS, a mother usually has results before she feels life and before a pregnancy is visible, a distinct advantage in being able to deal privately with any abnormality.

Both amniocentesis and CVS carry minimal risks of bleeding, infection, or miscarriage, but each is done with ultrasound guidance so that the doctor performing the procedure can see where his or her instruments are going. In 1991, reports began to surface that described an association between CVS and limb defects in infants. In 1989, blissfully unaware of such a risk, I counseled my sister to have a CVS with her first pregnancy at forty-two years of age. Thankfully, she gave birth to a healthy baby boy and now, over twenty years later, the newer CVS procedures are considered safer.

Maternal age-related risk for fetal chromosomal abnormalities is the most common reason to perform CVS or amniocentesis. However, we offer fetal testing to prospective mothers or fathers of any age when they have a family history of certain conditions. Fetal cells from amniotic fluid or placenta provide DNA for the diagnosis of hundreds of conditions, among them: cystic fibrosis, hemophilia, muscular dystrophy, and sickle cell disease.

Amniocentesis is useful as well to diagnose neural-tube defects. When the fetal spine fails to close over completely, a protein called alpha-fetoprotein (AFP) leaks out through the opening, and can be measured in the amniotic fluid. When a CVS is done instead of amniocentesis, AFP can be measured in the mother's blood. Then, if that level is elevated, an amniocentesis might be required for verification, or an ultrasound to visualize any abnormality.

Advanced paternal age (APA) carries some risks as well, but for single gene mutations. The "little person" with short limbs and a disproportionately large head is an Achondroplastic dwarf who was most likely born to an older father. APA is considered to be about forty-five years of age, but it is non-specific enough that our Division Chief, Dr. Ming-liang Lee jokingly defined it as, "one year older than I am."

In addition to tuning in to a patient's ability to absorb information, a genetic counselor must remain sensitive to different cultural nuances. That was singularly driven home to me, not by a patient, but by a colleague.

Ming-liang Lee is an MD/PhD trained in Taiwan. After completing a prestigious fellowship at Johns Hopkins Medical School with Dr. Victor McKusick, who is known as the "Father of Genetics," Dr. Lee became Division Chief of Genetics within the Department of Pediatrics at Rutgers Medical School. He is a brilliant and very caring man, but with a pragmatic efficiency of action, thought, and word.

Distraught one day over my father's worsening condition after his having suffered a stroke, I sought solace from Ming.

"How old is father?" he asked.

"Eighty-two," I answered.

"He already on borrowed time," was his clipped, accented consolation.

As Division Chief, Ming ultimately was responsible for overseeing my counseling practice, and he would soon give me even greater pause. A couple with two severely retarded sons had sought prenatal genetic counseling. The burden of this couple's struggle to care for two handicapped children seemed overwhelming. The woman, whom I'll call Ruth, wanted nothing more than to carry a normal, healthy child. If prenatal testing showed Ruth carried a girl, we could assure her that a daughter would, at worst, be an unaffected carrier.

Whereas an "autosomal" disease is inherited via one of the 22 non-sex chromosomes, a sex-linked disease, which Ruth's boys had, is inherited via the sex or X chromosome.

Females have two X chromosomes, whereas males have one X and a smaller Y. When a female inherits an abnormal mutation on an X from her mother, the normal X that her father contributed to make her a girl (note: dad *does* determine gender) usually masks the effect of that mutation so that she "carries," but is not affected by, the sex-linked disorder. A male who inherits that same mutation has no compensatory second X and will be affected by the disorder. A male or a female who does not inherit the mutation will be unaffected and cannot pass it on.

X-Linked recessive, carrier mother

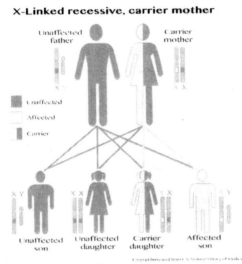

Researchers at the Institute for Basic Research (IBR) on Staten Island had just described new testing for the gene that caused Ruth's sons' retardation. The case became a teaching opportunity not only for members of our division, but also for the four or five residents who were rotating through our pediatrics department at the time.

Everyone working in our lab became vested in the couple's fate and a pall fell over the lab when the fetal cells were found to have a Y chromosome—it was a male. Because mom could have passed on either one of her two X chromosomes, we all hoped the little guy could still have inherited the gene from the mother's unaffected X chromosome.

Sadly, the testing showed the fetus to have the same gene as the two retarded boys. Because of the groundbreaking nature and teaching value of the case, we received permission from the couple to include two pediatric residents and a genetic counseling student in the session at which we delivered the results. I reserved a small conference room.

When the couple arrived, I had them wait in my office across the hall. I suspected that they could anticipate the results from my somber demeanor, yet they remained dignified in their distress. I escorted them into the conference room where seven pairs of eyes drilled into us. In a vain attempt to shield them, I seated them between Ming and me, with Ming positioned at the head of the table.

Ming would lead our discussion, Lenny review our laboratory results, and the researcher from IBR present their findings. Sitting across from our couple, he began explaining what his lab had found. It was a foregone conclusion that the couple would seek an abortion, as they had decided they were unable to care for three severely retarded boys. I saw before me a woman struggling to grasp the devastating news and beginning to mourn the healthy baby that she had hoped for. Because it was a new diagnosis at the time, it was important to obtain the couple's consent to get confirmatory samples from the aborted fetus.

Ming began addressing the entire conference room audience. "We will need to get a piece of the testes and a piece of liver from the abortus..." I recoiled at what seemed like a virtual dissection, as if the couple wasn't even in the room.

I slowly gathered my wits and interrupted him, "Ming, do we need to determine this now?"

"We probably could also use some brain...," he continued. His brain seemed to have switched into research mode, oblivious to this woman's carrying a living being that was still moving within her.

Horrified, I interrupted more forcefully, "I think this can wait!" I took Ruth's hand and headed for the door, her husband following. "I am so very sorry," I stammered.

"These things happen," her husband graciously assured me. Ruth seemed resolute and they left, hand in hand, with directions to the hospital where I was to meet them for the procedure in two days time.

All these years later, I still question my memory of that scene. Ming never acknowledged—at least to me—anything unusual about his behavior. I know he is not a cruel person, and I suspect his having reverted to a research mindset was a defense against his own anxiety.

Were I in the couple's place, I think that I would have been so angry and turned off that I would have wanted nothing at all to do with genetics, with the department, or with the entire medical school, but the following week I received a lovely flower arrangement from Ruth, with a note thanking me for my consideration. I wept at her kindness. I wept for her loss.

The interpersonal dynamics encountered while doing genetic counseling are fascinating to observe. Most common is blame. We have all heard snide comments in that blame game:

"That large head came from your father's side of the family!"

"You are acting just like your mother!"

"It was your Aunt Amy that brought this on our family!"

When someone is talking, not of a large head or annoying behavior, but of a serious disease, blame can fester and destroy. Combined with the stress of caring for a handicapped child, it can devastate even a solid relationship. The percentage of broken marriages increases two fold with the added stress of caring for a special-needs child, many of whose conditions have a genetic cause. The different inheritance patterns of diseases can lend themselves to predictable psychological responses.

X-linked Disorders

Just as with the retardation that affected Ruth's sons, the burden of guilt for an X-linked disorder falls to the mother who passed the disease to her sons. Russia's Empress Alexandra's guilt at having

68

passed hemophilia from her grandmother, Queen Victoria, to Prince Alexei, her only son and heir to the throne of Russia, made her vulnerable to the wiles of a Siberian peasant. A self-proclaimed holy man and healer, Rasputin was made a permanent figure in the royal court because Alexandra thought his prayers relieved her son's bleeding crises.

Tsar Nicholas II was unprepared to lead when he came to power at twenty-six. The ineffectual leadership of this anti-Semitic, autocratic ruler soon incited his people to revolt. When the Tsar went to the Eastern Front during World War I, Empress Alexandra increasingly ran the government and Rasputin grew in boldness, outrageous behavior, and influence in court.

Having decided that Rasputin's influence over the Tsaritsa had made him a threat to the empire, a group of nobles murdered Rasputin in December of 1916. With supplies exhausted and regiments beginning to mutiny, Nicholas held fast his crown. Three months after Rasputin's death, however, Nicholas was forced to abdicate amidst socialist parties vying for power. The subsequent Bolshevik revolution led to the infamous massacre of twenty members of the royal family. Thus, a single gene played a contributing role in the downfall of the three-hundred-year-old Romanov dynasty.

Shortly after seeing Ruth, I counseled a woman whom I will call Sara. Sara had several retarded maternal uncles, several retarded great uncles, and a retarded brother—a classic pattern of inheritance seen in X-linked disorders. Like Ruth, Sara decided on prenatal testing. We found that she was a carrier, and that her unborn son had inherited the retardation-causing gene.

Sara had been raised in a loving home with simple Christian values that harkened back to a time when people accepted the bad with the good, all of it "willed by God." Her retarded brother, Tommy, was central to the household, tenderly supported, and revered for the good nature and loyalty he gave his family, despite his limitations. Tommy's IQ was high enough that he had painful awareness of his own difficulties. "I can't do what all the other kids do," he told me with a resolute sadness in his voice.

During one of my visits to their home Tommy's cat had just had kittens. A little orange male looked exactly like one I had just lost, so Tommy insisted I take his kitten. I periodically sent Tommy pictures of "Boo" over the course of the cat's long and peaceful life with my family. Boo was a warm and fuzzy reminder of the bond that I had with the people whose lives I shared so intimately. He reminded me, too, of the hopes and fears that we all have in common.

Sara elected to have an abortion rather than to bring another male into the world to suffer as Tommy had. In an act of love that I felt privileged to witness, their mother stood fast by her daughter's decision. "It's not been bad having Tommy," the mother confided to me during one visit. "He's a loving person and he gives so much to us. Look at this picture taken of him with Governor Kean. Tommy was so proud to have his photo taken with the governor."

I think that Sara's mother simply would have accepted the birth of another affected male as "God's will." The technology that provided her daughter with alternative options must have transported her to unfamiliar, very frightening emotional territory, but she sat close by her daughter's side throughout the entire ordeal. More than 20 years later, the recollection of her generosity and selflessness fills me with admiration.

Dominant Disorders

Dominant disorders are passed vertically from generation to generation. It takes just one gene to cause the disease, so that each child of an affected parent has a straightforward 50% chance of being similarly affected, whether male or female.

Because the "responsible" side of the family is usually known, the blame game can become rampant. Working with several late-onset neurological diseases, I saw a spectrum of responses to a disease in which each child of an affected parent has a 50% chance of being similarly affected. With these conditions, the beginning of symptoms usually occurs after one has had children and already passed on the fateful gene.

Autosomal dominant

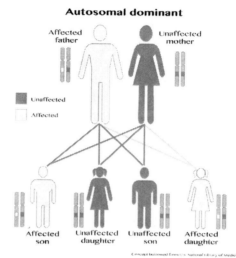

Imagine that your spouse's mother begins to lose the ability to control movement. You journey from doctor to doctor to find out why. You finally learn that her diagnosis is Huntington disease. You also learn that her future will only get worse. She likely will lose the ability to control her behavior, as well as the ability to think and reason. Imagine learning also that your spouse has a 50% chance of developing the same disorder. Lastly, imagine the devastation upon learning that, if your spouse does develop the disorder, the two of you may already have inadvertently passed the disease gene on to your children.

I have witnessed some people's open, loving acceptance after obtaining such information, adopting a "we're in this together" spirit. I also have seen HD families blown apart by the secrecy surrounding this diagnosis. One woman I counseled was literally told about HD on the night before her wedding. Her well-meaning family members finally decided, presumably lest she get pregnant, that it was time to tell her that the strange disease which left her father flailing, half delirious, and ranting in an asylum was called Huntington disease. And, by the way, she had a 50% chance of being similarly affected. She was afraid of losing her husband-to-be, so the wedding

71

proceeded without informing him, and she bore the guilt of deception. Her husband remained blissfully unaware of the waiting pyre until she began developing symptoms years later. Had she forewarned her fiancé about her father, her own diagnosis might have marked the renewal of support and devotion; instead, her husband was forced to grapple simultaneously with his wife's diagnosis and a long-standing breach of trust. Recalling this today can fill me with sadness at the realization of what hurt can be wrought in the name of love, what pain delivered on the wings of secrecy.

Recessive Disorders

These are more egalitarian. Because it takes a gene from each parent to cause a recessive disorder, one observes less of the blame game and more of a shared sadness in the discovery that two partners just happened to mate with someone who carried a mutation, or change, in the same gene.

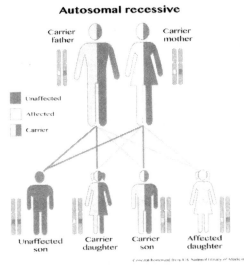

Autosomal recessive

When people got caught up in the word, "abnormal," I always emphasized that not one of us is truly normal. Each one of us has some seven or eight genes with arbitrary mutations that are capable of causing a recessive disease if we partnered with someone who also had a defect in that same gene. Having an increased number of shared genes raises the likelihood of that happening. That is why recessive disorders can be found among offspring from a union between closely related individuals.

Lest it seem that everything in clinical genetics is doom and gloom, let me tell you about one success story. I had the opportunity to counsel a pregnant woman, whom I will dub Lila, with cystic fibrosis (CF). This bubbly young woman had an identical twin, Laura, who, because the two shared all of their genes, also had CF. In and of itself, their existence was miraculous, because many CF kids don't make it through to adulthood, never mind carry a pregnancy. Lila's mom accompanied her to our meeting and told me of the typical CF "rescue": her constantly having to slap both kids' backs to loosen their chest congestion. When Lila became pregnant she and her mom were very worried about the possibility of recurrence in her baby.

Because CF is recessive, Lila's baby would not be affected unless Lila's husband, to whom she was not related, also happened to carry a mutation in the CF gene. The chances were slim and blood testing confirmed that his CF gene was indeed free of known mutations. Lila and Laura had inherited one affected CF gene from their mother and one from their father. But, as long as Lila or Laura's mates were non-carriers, all their children would be, at worst, healthy carriers. Through genetic counseling, family members learned that they could avoid having to deal with CF in subsequent generations. Because of her own CF Lila required careful, high-risk obstetric care throughout her pregnancy, but she delivered a perfect little version of herself—a version without CF.

A few short months later, I received a photo in the mail of a very happy looking Lila holding her precious, little, blond baby girl. Accompanying the photo was a note, "Thanks, Aunt Alice, for helping to make my mommy so happy."

Chapter X

THE HUNTINGTON'S DISEASE FAMILY SERVICE CENTER

In 1978, I became aware of a new statewide program being developed for Huntington disease. Two men, each of whom had an immense impact on my professional life, initiated the program. I luxuriated in their accolades during the eleven years that I worked with HD families.

The first was my mentor, Mike McCormack. Though nine years my junior, in some ways Mike reminded me of my dad—he had class and charm, a shock of red hair, and an Irish twinkle in his eye. His natural charisma and his PhD in Medical Genetics allowed him to parlay his connections with New Jersey's State Department of Health to considerable funding advantage and to offer New Jersey residents genetic services.

In 1975, the gene for sickle cell anemia had recently been found. Mike and I, and everyone in the field of genetics, knew that we were on the brink of finding cures for diseases that had baffled generations before us. I had taken compulsive notes in Mike's class in biochemical genetics. I was awed when he said he developed a potential cure for sickle cell disease, and I fed the novel idea right back to him on an exam. It would not be the last time that my attention to detail served me well, nor would it be the last time Mike voiced his encouragement to me: "Alice, you are one of the smartest people in the genetic counseling program. You really should go on and get your PhD."

The second man was Samuel L Baily. Sam, a graduate of Harvard University, had been steeped in a strong Quaker heritage. I came to admire greatly and to learn from the erudition that Sam managed to combine with his principled and generous way of life. To me, Sam personified the Christian ideals that I had been taught and to which I aspired. He did not preach, but taught by his example. Sam's mother had had HD, so that he was at 50% risk of developing the disorder. Sam was a doer, an eloquent professor of history, and an active member of the lay organization for HD who used his gift with words to advocate tirelessly for HD families. When Marjorie Guthrie's Committee to Combat Huntington's Disease (CCHD) and the National Huntington's Disease Association (NHDA), eventually merged into the current Huntington's Disease Society of America (HDSA), Sam choreographed the merger.

Sam had been contacted by a man, desperate to find help for his wife who suffered from end stage HD. Never one to let another's need go unanswered, Sam approached Mike for aid in establishing a program to which HD family members might come for services. The combination of Sam's selfless dedication and Mike's political connections to persons directing state funding for genetics soon made support for the program a reality.

In 1979 the Huntington's Disease Family Service Center (HDFSC) opened in New Jersey, and I had secured the position as its coordinator. The center was later officially named the Samuel L. Baily Huntington's Disease Family Service Center, in honor of its founder. Lenny, Mike, and others in the Genetic Counseling program had given me glowing recommendations, but I like to think that my commitment to HD and my people skills also were evident. I think, too, that there is a guiding force—something that takes us down one pathway and not another—and I was meant to take the path that I took in helping HD families.

We set up a multidisciplinary center staffed by neurology, psychiatry, neuropsychology, rehabilitative medicine, and genetics personnel, and held regularly scheduled clinics in which patients and families partook of the different disciplines depending on their needs. As coordinator, I served as both genetic counselor and social worker. New Jersey's Family Service Center soon became a model for service provision for Huntington's families, and other HDSA chapters throughout the country adopted our lead and hired at least a part-time social worker. The years I spent coordinating the HDFSC were fulfilling years. I was making a difference in many ways.

Our HDFSC was funded by "soft" money, that is, money from whatever grants Mike was able to cobble together each year. Mike made me acutely aware that funding—and my job—could disappear. I am fairly sure Mike was aware that my family was dependent on my health insurance and on my salary. Still, every year at funding time we reenacted a familiar script.

"Alice, I'm not sure we can pick up your salary next year."

I simply rolled my eyes and grimaced. Then I took my private panic home.

My God, what are we going to do? became my mantra as my children approached the age at which they would attend college. I had witnessed Mike axe his friend, Ann, and had commiserated with her about the injustice of it all. I lived in constant fear that he might do the same to me.

Bob reassured me, "Alice, Mike genuinely likes you. You take his teasing too seriously."

Over the years, Mike probably had his own real concerns for the future of our program, and his job as its director. I believed it was my tenacity and my relationship with HD family members that was the heart and soul of our HDFSC program, yet I was acutely aware that Mike's expertise in the financial aspects of our program made him the more fit in the Darwinian sense. If funding demands should force us to downsize, reducing the program to the survival of the fittest, it was clear to me that I was the more dispensable. Despite my fears, Mike did manage to continue funding my position.

🕊

One day a former high-powered New York broker named Dennis Shea came into my office with a painful story about his wife's HD. Dennis had light blue eyes that seemed to reflect the vast blue sky, and he had an equally enormous determination to change the face of HD research. Financially sound, he had retired early and taken up a new career. He was determined to use his many high rolling former colleagues and contacts to raise money for HD, and he had the charm to persuade them to help his cause.

Dennis constantly voiced his appreciation at my having been there when he needed information and support. I could hear Mike's financial antennae vibrating in response. To Mike, those accolades translated into potential support of our HDFSC. But, while Dennis valued our program of service, he had children at risk of developing the disorder. He was clearly more vested in funding research to find a cure, and Dennis had the wherewithal to pursue his dream.

In 1986, just a few short months after we had met, he phoned me at my office. "Alice. I'm putting together a foundation for HD, and I want you to be on the advisory board, along with Nancy Wexler and several of my bond guys from Wall Street. We'll raise lots of money for research and find the cure."

He didn't ask Mike—he asked me!

"That sounds quite ambitious, and very exciting," I said, trying to keep my voice nonchalant and professional.

"Can you make a meeting next Friday night? Nancy is in town and Frank can fly up from Florida. I'll send a limo to pick you up and we'll meet at the University Club in New York. Eight o'clock?"

A limo. For me!

"Sure, Friday will work."

I had never sat on a board advising anything. I felt honored. Here was someone who so valued my input regarding the disposition of

78

monies for research, that he would send a limousine to pick me up for meetings in New York City. In 1989 Dennis's Foundation for the Care and Cure of Huntington's Disease held a fundraiser featuring the former Nobel laureate James Watson as honored guest. We raised over $1,000,000 in that one evening for HD research, much of which we channeled into Jim Gusella's research program at Massachusetts General Hospital.

I had met Jim Gusella in 1983 while attending a meeting of the American Society of Human Genetics in Boston. One session went late into the night. After back-to-back meetings all day, participants are usually saturated with new information and begin to doze off. But this night was different. The genetics research community had heard word that something really big was breaking.

A slightly rotund, be-speckled, and very young looking man named Jim Gusella neared the podium, but turned the presentation over to his graduate fellow, Marcy MacDonald. Speaking in a soft, unassuming voice she began, "Huntington's disease is an autosomal dominant, late-onset neurological disorder, characterized by the inability to control extraneous, dance-like movements, by cognitive loss, as well as by psychiatric manifestations..."After her introduction, she went on to the other prescribed sections of a scientific presentation: materials and methods, then results. "We have identified a marker on chromosome 4p that segregates with the HD gene...," she announced.

DNA 'markers' are small pieces of DNA that show normal variations between people and have been mapped throughout the chromosomes. They may have no particular significance but, if a disease-causing gene just happens to be located near one of these markers, they will be inherited together. By charting the inheritance of known markers through affected and unaffected members of HD families, Gusella and his team had located the HD gene on the short arm of chromosome number four! The crowd erupted. I stood. Everyone stood. We applauded and cheered wildly.

Three years earlier, gene mapping technology had been reported which would enable researchers to determine the location of a gene (its "locus" on a chromosome). The HD gene was the first to be mapped using this new "linkage mapping." It had been estimated that it would require more than three hundred detailed genetic analyses, each taking weeks to perform, in order to determine the whereabouts of that gene, but they had located it on the twelfth try!

"Jim," as I was privileged to call him, had achieved a landmark in the field of genetics. I, and many others, thought that his breakthrough might very well earn him a Nobel Prize. To congratulate Jim, I sent him a bottle of wine with a bottle cover that I had "dressed" as a huntsman—replete with scarlet coat, riding cap, horn, and a banner that read, "HD Gene Hunt." Thirteen years later, I would also present wine-bottle huntsmen with banners reading "PD Gene Hunt" to my fellow Parkinson disease huntsmen.

After the excitement of locating *where* the HD gene was, came the frustration of determining *what* the gene was. Researchers had to span the genetic distance from the marker and close in on the actual gene. Because the HD gene happened to be in an area that was particularly difficult to study, and the science back then was in its infancy, it took another ten long years to do this. In 1993 the HD-causing gene was identified and named "IT15" (important transcript 15) and later "huntingtin."

Alas, research can be painfully slow, and Dennis Shea did not live to see all that has ensued from his inspired generosity. At the age of fifty-five, he succumbed to cancer, but anyone familiar with his contribution will tell you that a cure is far closer than it would have been without the efforts of the man whom I had dubbed, "HD's ol' blue eyes."

When the location of the causative gene for HD was determined in 1983, it became technically feasible to determine if an at-risk person likely carried a faulty HD gene. The way we did this was by seeing whether their affected parent passed on the DNA markers that Jim Gusella had found were very near to the HD gene. If a person carried the same markers as their affected parent, he or she most likely carried the faulty HD gene along with those markers.

Until such predictive testing became available the only option for someone who was at 50% risk of developing HD to avoid passing on the disease was to refrain from having children. Many professionals considered it downright selfish of persons who knew they were at risk to chance passing the gene to the next generation. "People at risk should just not have children," was crusaded in the literature.

If you think about it, however, choosing to not have children in that situation is an acknowledgement that there really is a problem with this HD thing and it might happen to you. On the other hand having children—"normalizing," if you will—is an effective way to deny that reality and to send yourself the message that it might happen to the other guy, but it won't happen to you.

HD families and activists had been very eager to have options, so that when the gene was localized in 1983, they began to pressure the professional community of neurologists, counselors and geneticists to make testing available. In order that they might more realistically plan their future, people who lived with the uncertainty of a 50% risk wanted to be tested and to learn whether their risk was closer to 0% (meaning that they likely did not carry the faulty gene) or if it was closer to 100% (which meant they likely did carry the gene). However, between 1983 and 1993, when the actual gene was identified, predictive testing was only about 90 to 95% accurate. An error rate of 5 to 10% in predicting that one would develop such an utterly devastating disease could have profoundly dangerous effects, including suicide. Since there was no cure, a positive test result by itself was likened by many to a "prolonged death sentence."

I was involved with the HD community in developing standards for how to administer this predictive testing. I was honored to have my opinion about a key development in my field sought by my peers. Early on, it was decided not to test minors, to require screening by a psychiatrist to assess emotional stability, and to have a third party present as an extra set of ears throughout the counseling. Together we developed a comprehensive eight-session program of screening and counseling for persons at-risk for HD who requested predictive testing. In questionnaires that we administered before the HD gene was localized, about half of at-risk individuals declared intend to be tested. Once Jim Gusella's breakthrough made testing feasible, only about 10% of persons actually requested testing.

Telling someone with great certainty that they will develop a disease that will so cruelly rob them of their dignity was the most sobering task I have ever undertaken. It was one that I felt privileged to be trusted with, but one that brought with it an awesome responsibility for the well being of another. I could not have done it without my professional colleagues at our HDFSC.

At about the same time that predictive testing became available, we were able to bring on board a licensed social worker, Rhoda Grossman. A strikingly pretty, middle-aged woman with brown eyes and full-bodied, dark, curly hair, her soft voice transmitted a calm caring to each patient or family member with whom she interacted, as well as to her fellow professionals. I was initially resistant to a social worker coming into my program. I felt threatened that her social worker training made her better able to fulfill the needs of our families and that she might replace me if funding became tight. However, Rhoda conveyed respect for the relationship that I had established with our families and, valuing what I contributed, she quickly made me feel at ease. Rhoda helped me to hone my ability to empathize with those in pain and to help them feel that they were not alone. Together we formed a team, each augmenting the other. We both felt humbled by the responsibility that had been thrust upon us as caretakers to the very souls of our patients. After each heavily-laden predictive testing session, we debriefed, sometimes for hours, but always together. I was immensely relieved to have someone with whom to share this daunting task.

Doing predictive testing for HD, I repeatedly was struck by the power of denial. The main reason at-risk persons requested testing was to plan for the future. This implied that, if one knew for certain whether he or she carried the gene, one would do things differently. Sometimes this future plan involved decisions about career choice or life style: whether to invest in prolonged job training, say, to be a surgeon if one had only a few good years in which to practice, or whether to do something one could enjoy immediately. Frequently it involved decisions about procreation: whether to bring children into the world who might watch a parent deteriorate, then possibly develop the disease him or herself.

I will call one couple that came to us requesting predictive testing, Joan and Harry. They had had several children before Joan's mother was diagnosed with HD, a life-altering trauma for the entire family. With her mother's diagnosis, Joan immediately became at 50% risk for developing HD, and each of her children, at 25% risk. The couple learned of the availability of predictive testing, and decided that, if Joan were tested and found to be negative, they might have more children; if she were positive, they would not. A bright, reflective, devoted couple, together they constituted the ideal candidates for our new predictive testing program. They regularly attended each of our required counseling sessions and passed the screening with flying colors—no psychiatric red flags, a clear understanding of the implications of testing, a realistic acceptance of the possibility that Joan could be identified as a gene-carrier, and a recognition that once given, the results could not be taken back.

Shortly before our scheduled disclosure session, our team got the results from the laboratory that Joan carried her mother's gene markers, and would most likely develop HD. Rhoda and I were devastated for the couple, and had to convey the sad news to them. After ushering them into our tiny conference room, I said, "Joan, the laboratory results show that you carry the same HD gene markers as your mother. I am so sorry to have to tell you this, when each of us had hoped for different news."

Rhoda reached across the table to take each of their hands in hers and said softly, "I am so very sorry." She paused, and then continued, "Alice and I will remain available for whatever the two of you may need."

Rhoda and I then waited in quiet sadness, letting Joan and Harry absorb what they perhaps had read in our body language even as we first greeted them. When they had no immediate questions, we excused ourselves to let them have some private time together.

83

When we came back, eyes were teary—theirs and ours. During hours of counseling we had come to know them intimately: their dreams and fears, their hope that they might be spared this sentencing, their desire to have another child without the specter of HD looming. In that one moment, HD was no longer a remote possibility, but their very future.

It was done. They needed to leave, to get away from the place of sadness, and away from the messengers of bad news. We made sure they had our emergency contact numbers and told them we would call to follow up with them within the next twenty-four hours. Now it was theirs to process how to integrate this new information into their lives.

We kept in regular contact over the next few weeks to assure that they were handling the information as well as could be expected. After several months passed, I received a phone call from Joan.

"Alice, I've got news. Harry and I are pregnant."

At first I was surprised. Her news stood in stark contrast to her stated intent prior to learning she carried the HD gene. Then I realized how consistent her response was with the denial I had observed—another stab at normalizing. Going about life as usual is a refusal to allow entry to the monster.

This need to keep the monster at bay would one day take on a very personal urgency for me.

Chapter XI
PHILADELPHIA FREEDOM

March 1985

Just before St. Patrick's Day Mike had announced that he was leaving UMDNJ-Robert Wood Johnson Medical School in New Brunswick and affiliating the Huntington's Disease Family Service Center with its sister school, UMDNJ-School of Osteopathic Medicine in Camden. Not only was Mike relocating the HD program, to which I had devoted myself for the past six years, but I saw my very livelihood being jeopardized.

Mike must have seen through to my panic. I think, too, he knew how highly the HD families regarded me, and he valued my contribution to the program. "Why don't you come with me to Camden?" he offered.

Feeling instantly reckless with his possible reprieve, I retorted, "You'd have to make it worth my while to commute the two hours from North Jersey and afford an apartment to stay in during the week."

He did, and I did, and my Huntington's work extended another five years.

I rented the upper two floors of a red brick trinity in the Society Hill section of Philadelphia. A short commute across the Ben Franklin Bridge and I was at work in Camden. Trinities, in Philadelphia parlance, are three story houses built between 1790 and 1840.

Generally one room per floor, their name was homage to the Father, Son and Holy Ghost.

I was forty-five. It was my first taste of living alone. I liked it...a lot. I called that apartment my "yuppie pad," to which my mother gently pointed out, "Alice, you're too old to be a yuppie."

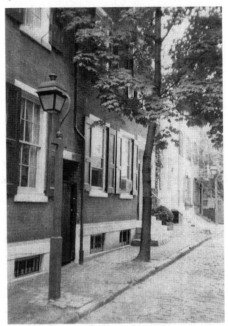

300 South American Street

When my daughter Kathi applied to medical school, she was accepted first into Tufts, but that would have meant her going to Boston. When she got into the University of Pennsylvania Medical School, and we learned that the tuition there was $2,000 less per year, our sharing the Philadelphia apartment became a logical arrangement. She already had lived independently as an undergraduate at Rutgers, so she was willing to share living quarters with her mother. On the weekends, Kathi's future husband, Paul, came down from New York City and I headed back to home, and husband, in North Jersey in order to wash and restock my clothes.

Bob visited only occasionally while Kathi and I were living in Philly. When offered an invitation, he clearly preferred to stay by himself. I, on the other hand, thoroughly enjoyed the opportunity to buy season tickets to the ballet and invite friends to join me to hear the Philadelphia Orchestra, to entertain at leisure. There was a clear message, had I listened to it, that I could do just fine on my own. I was more relaxed, and indeed, happier.

Our trinity had four levels and was rather generous in size. We had a living room and kitchen on the first level and two bedrooms on the second. Since we had only the upper two floors of the house, we didn't have direct access to the tiny backyard garden patio, but from our kitchen window we looked out over the sweetest pink dogwood tree. Behind the patio was a gated parking area where my designated spot welcomed me at the end of a long day at work. I had only to walk around a short block to the cobblestone alleyway leading to our front door.

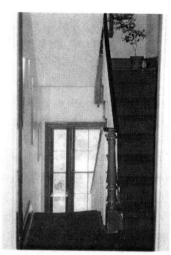

Our apartment's stairs

Moving in was a bit of a challenge. I had ordered a modestly priced sofa without regard for the narrow, twisting stairs, but the deliverymen somehow managed to maneuver it in. There were copious built-in bookcases and a fireplace in each bedroom, so that I was able to make it cozy with only a few other items from home: a stereo and second TV provided the living-room entertainment, a glass-top table and ice-cream parlor chairs serviced our tiny eat-in kitchen, and my son's long-forgotten twin bed served me just fine. Kathi decorated her room with a king-size waterbed, neither one of us considering the possible consequences if it should ever leak.

Sharing that apartment with my daughter was one of the most treasured experiences of my life. Because there were just the two of us, we were less like mother and daughter, and more like roommates. I saw a more relaxed, self-assured daughter, one happy to find things we could do together.

"Mom, why don't we go down to the secondhand bookstore on South Street after supper?"

"Mom, do you feel like Thai food tonight?"

"Mom, if you stay here this weekend we could go to the Penn Street Festival."

"Mom, when I graduate could we go to the Marrakesh Moroccan restaurant?" She chuckled, "I want to see Dad eat with his hands."

During the four years we lived in Philly together, Kathi and I both kept busy schedules. Still, we managed to find time to soak up some of Philly's history. We never established if we were related to Francesco Lazzarini, but we delighted in discovering that he had sculpted the marble statue of Benjamin Franklin that sits in the arched niche above the Library Company's door. Then, we saw Ben himself walking the city street—an actor, of course, but buoyed by the quaint brick buildings, the street lanterns, and cobblestone streets, believably real.

I brought my bike to Philly, and Kathi and I rode down Benjamin Franklin Parkway and up Kelly drive, winding along the Schuylkill River, past Boathouse Row and Fairmount Park. One evening found us sitting on the lawn at the Mann Center, sipping wine together and watching the Bolshoi Ballet as the Philadelphia lights twinkled in the distance.

Strolling through picturesque back alleyways to the market on Fifth Street off Chestnut in order to restock our larder was a wonderful opportunity to hear about her experiences. She told me of the prank she and two anatomy-class partners contrived when they had lost patience with their sloppy bench mate, Albert. "We rigged our cadaver to sit up on command and emit a recorded message, 'Clean up Albert.' I thought Albert was gonna shit a brick when that half-dissected body talked to him," she guffawed.

"I've been chosen to be the surgeon for the class photograph of The Agnew Clinic for our school calendar," she boasted one day. Thomas Eakins' famous painting, "The Agnew Clinic," was commissioned in 1889 by a group of students to honor Dr. Agnew

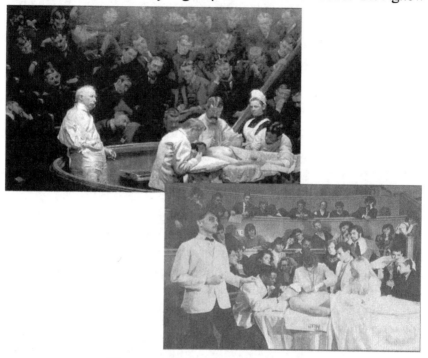

Thomas Eakins's The Agnew Clinic

on his retirement. Once prominently featured in the medical school's main academic building, it is now on permanent loan to the Philadelphia Museum of Art. I have the staged, calendar version prominently featured in my office.

While in Philly, I bore witness to Kathi's metamorphosis from a carefree college grad into a caring physician. I treasure the memory of her excitement upon getting her first white coat. But, the day she came home with her first stethoscope and tried to listen to my heart, she suddenly blanched.

"What's wrong?" I ventured.

She had not been able to find my heart. "Don't worry, Mom, you have one somewhere," she reassured, and we both laughed.

Even as she studied, Kathi managed to learn how to bake shiny bakery-worthy loaves of bread and how to knit cable sweaters that looked as though they came straight from an Irish knit shop. One day I came home to find Kathi leaning over our bathtub trying to wash mites out of ears that looked bigger than the body of the scrawny kitten who owned them.

"Isn't he the cutest thing you've ever seen?" she exclaimed.

Not exactly!

Tigger grew into a cat with such a large appetite that we had to bolt the cabinet containing the garbage pail. He once pulled a corncob from the garbage disposal with his paw, and we had to take him to the vet's in order to 'dis-impact' his bowel.

Then came the even "cuter" baby boa constrictor, Gerry. Gerry's food came from the pet store—alive. First it was mice. The transport box read, "Congratulations. You have found a good home." *Right!* Gerry then moved up to rats. Another day I came home to find Gerry in my bed; Kathi had just given her a bath. "Mom, I won't be much longer. My waterbed jiggles, so your bed is a better place for me to dry her off."

"Whatever," I said. Feeling queasy, I turned and left to put distance between the squirmy reptile and me. Gerry lived in Kathi's room in an aquarium with a wire screen top where Tigger perched. As Gerry grew, I shut Kathi's bedroom door whenever I passed her room. I didn't want to witness Gerry's move up to cats! Tigger and Gerry were definitely Kathi's. Neither would have been my choice for a roommate, but I took great pleasure in seeing Kathi's happiness in such simple, everyday things.

Tigger survived, but Gerry had to be given away when, at about six-feet in length, she got her jaws around Kathi's arm. I'm just grateful that it wasn't Gerry's body around Kathi's neck! Kathi was appalled that her beloved Gerry turned on her, but she wound up donating her pet to the Franklin Institute. The friend who accompanied Kathi on that altruistic mission via public transportation, often relayed the embarrassment she felt as Kathi repeatedly wailed, "I can't believe I'm giving my baby away." Once Kathi got over her grief, we laughed together at the spectacle she must have made.

Doing clinical rounds in her third year of medical school, Kathi rejected each specialty—until she found radiology. "Mom, I can't believe they're going to pay me to do this!" It was the same way I felt about genetics, and I knew she had found her passion. That was the year she had met Paul at a friend's wedding. "Mom, he's just like my brother," she had burst in with excitement, "so smart and easy to be with." And, I knew she had also found her love.

Now, every time I recall these memories and so many, many more, I think of her beautiful face, and I smile.

In 1990, when Kathi graduated from medical school, she accepted an internship at Morristown Memorial Hospital some ten miles from my North Jersey home. That same year Roger Duvoisin, Chairman of Neurology at UMDNJ-RWJMS in New Brunswick, NJ, recruited me to join the team that he was forming as part of his department's new William Dow Lovett Center for Neurogenetics. It would mean giving up my HD work. It would also mean relocating back to New Brunswick.

I had coordinated the HD Family Service Center for eleven years, five years living in Philadelphia and commuting home on weekends. I was fond of the HD families with whom I worked, but I was stressed from sharing their never-ending heartbreak. Even from my current vantage point, having studied many different neurological disorders, and having been diagnosed with one of my own, Huntington stands out as one of the cruelest. The child of an HD patient looks at an affected parent and sees the specter of his or her own demise. I was even starting to see the children of some of my patients develop the disease.

The location of the Huntington disease gene had been mapped to chromosome number four in 1983, but by 1990 the gene itself still had not been identified. Locating the general whereabouts of a gene was like looking for a house, finding its town, but not knowing the address of the house, or what that house looked like. Waiting for that house to be identified, I was finding it increasingly difficult to remain upbeat and maintain the positive outlook that was required to help my HD families.

Kathi and I had shared memorable times as roommates in Philly but, as she moved on, so did I. I would miss the freedom and independence of my yuppie pad, but I realized that I could not continue my weekend commute to North Jersey indefinitely. Besides, if I were back in North Jersey, I could continue spending time with Kathi and Paul.

I accepted Roger's offer, and in October of 1990, packed up my apartment and said a teary goodbye to my adopted city of Philadelphia.

Chapter XII
YOU CAN GO HOME AGAIN

"I'll be retiring long before you do. Will you be okay with that?" Roger Duvoisin asked me over lunch. He had invited me for a pro forma interview in the faculty dining room, and was expressing concern for my staying power once he retired and could no longer protect me.

"No problem," I answered. "I can get along just fine with anyone," I boasted, rather flippantly.

Roger's dark eyes and eyebrows contrasted sharply with a thick head of pure white hair. A tall man in his sixties and dressed in a conservative suit and tie, he exuded class. He was thirteen years my senior, but I was sure his enthusiasm for science was not going to allow him to step down anytime soon.

"I need a geneticist. I need you," he told me, his eyes bright with excitement. "I'm sure I can continue the faculty position you've had by appointing you Assistant Professor."

I was flattered that he chose me to be part of his department's new research venture. "Tell me what you envision me doing," I asked.

After explaining the nature of my new responsibilities, he continued, "I'd like you to sit on the search committee we'll put together to find a medical director."

His faith in me superseded any apprehension that I might have had over such high expectations. His respectful manner made me feel comfortable that I could trust him with a major shift in my career. By the time we said goodbye, I knew I was destined to move back home.

Roger's Department of Neurology had received a $3.5 million endowment, the largest in the history of the medical school. Roger was an astute observer of his patients and their families and knew that genetics was the key to understanding the many devastating neurological diseases that he and his colleagues struggled to treat. With the endowment, he was able to establish the William Dow Lovett Laboratory for Neurogenetics in which to do research and contribute to that understanding.

Like my dad, Roger's father had taught at Parsons School of Design. Roger told me that his father had illustrated children's books, one of them about a goose named Petunia. If you do a book search on "Roger Duvoisin," it will yield books on both "Petunia" (the father's) and "Parkinson disease" (the son's). I stood in awe of this man's professional accomplishments, and was surprised to learn that his artist father had actually discouraged his becoming a physician.

Roger had become Chairman of the Department of Neurology at what was then Rutgers Medical School in 1979, the same year that we had started the Huntington's Disease Family Service Center (HDFSC). At the HDFSC, we had had professionals from other disciplines, among them genetics and psychiatry, but we depended on Roger to appoint a neurologist to participate in our HD clinic. Over the years he had observed my work on behalf of Huntington disease patients, and he knew of my passion for genetics.

A Columbia trained neurologist with a career-long devotion to Parkinson's research and patients, Roger wrote the classic, *Parkinson's Disease, A Guide for Patient and Family.* He began his career as a Navy corpsman, enlisting in WWII before he finished high school. Upon discharge he completed college and medical school, and after residency, served four years in the Neurology Service at Lackland Air Force Hospital in San Antonio, Texas. In 1962 Dr. H. Houston Merritt offered him an appointment at Columbia's Neurological Institute. Merritt, who had authored Merritt's Textbook of Neurology, was affectionately known as "The Boss." Out of respect and admiration, Merritt's tradition was carried on, and Roger also became known to his faculty as "The Boss."

🕊

My new venture had such an aura of excitement that I felt anything was possible. I could commute to New Brunswick from my home in North Jersey and once again lived full time with Bob. Living and managing on my own in Philadelphia, however, had given me a new self-assurance. Simply knowing that I could do it made me more tolerant of any day-to-day difficulties in my marriage, a bit like having a car in your driveway—just knowing it's there gives you a sense of freedom, even if you choose not to use it. I chose not to use it. The salary increase I had parlayed in going to Camden, along with relief from the costs of an apartment and of tuition bills, provided a financial cushion for the first time in our lives. So, too, the freedom from packing and moving on a weekly basis was a great relief.

I worked full days, coming home with just enough time to have a bit of dinner and retire for the night. I contributed the maximum to my retirement plan. I worked even more. I got season tickets to the Metropolitan Opera. I worked more. Bob and I got in some traveling together. He had initiated some mood-stabilizing medication, and with just the two of us, the time we did spend together seemed improved.

🕊

Saying goodbye to my adopted HD family was difficult. On February 10, 1991, I was thrown a "thank you" party (I had stipulated that I did not "do" goodbyes). By then, I had already made the transition to Roger's department, so the get together was a joyous opportunity to see dear friends and colleagues again and to share their accolades with my family.

I had not seen Jackie, the friend who had inspired my work with HD, in some time. Then, as I was circulating amongst my friends I saw her slip unobtrusively into the entranceway. I had been too busy to keep in touch recently, and yet she had driven over an hour to honor me.

I smiled and walked toward her, then halted. I saw that she was now moving in an unmistakable dance-like way. My gut clenched as it railed against what I was seeing, and I fought to contain my horror. My strong, invincible friend, my "Captain Sunshine," had fallen victim to this Goddamned cruel disease. She seemed unaware of her movements—and their portent. My delight was now tinged with sadness, and I struggled to strike a casual air in welcoming her to the festive celebration. Realizing that she now had HD only validated the appropriateness of my decision to move on. I no longer took care of the multitudes with HD, but I would be able to have quality time for a few, very special HD patients.

As I look now through a memento album that was put together for the occasion, I still am touched as I read praise for my having "offered hope, humanity and compassion," and for "having been central in the development and flourishing of a center that is a model for the country." I see myself in photographs with happy summer campers, on one of the many bike rides we took to raise money for HD, and accepting an award from HD's ol' blue eyes, Dennis Shea.

Then my eyes tear up as I read a note from the mother of my very first HD patient. Linda's mom thanked me for sharing lunches and laughs with her daughter, and for bringing Linda red roses when she turned forty, already quite impaired by HD. When Linda came into my office in 1979 at twenty-nine years of age, her modeling was over and her job as a secretary was already in jeopardy from the ravages of HD. I did not bring all my patients birthday roses, but I cared deeply for each of them.

"You have a wonderful way of connecting with people," remarked a psychologist with whom I once led an HD support group. I still take great pride in her compliment, and credit that ability with my success in working with HD families. I think it boiled down to conveying a sense of, "you can trust me because I'm right in there with you."

I pray that all those years of being right in there with my patients will afford me the grace that I will need to let others care for me when the time comes.

Chapter XIII
ATAXIA IS NOT A FOREIGN CAB

William Dow Lovett, Billy (or "Beellee" as his wife, with her deep southern drawl, called him) had a kind of ataxia, or loss of muscle control. He owned a well-known food chain in the South and, in the late 1980's, he periodically flew from Florida to New Jersey's Robert Wood Johnson Medical School in order to see neurologist Margery Mark for treatment.

Although separated by years, Margery and Billy had both attended Yale. He used to say that her unique blend of forthrightness and irreverence, her strong will and good humor, as well as her clinical competence made him a devotee. Billy resolved to endow a research university to help find a gene for the ataxia that was affecting his balance and limiting his ability to walk. His trust in Margery, and no doubt their both being "Yalies," contributed to his generosity to the neurology department.

Our team's hunt was on for the gene(s) causing *ataxia*.

Roger asked me to identify and construct family histories of persons with ataxia who were seen in our neurology clinic. While Billy Lovett's family was not large enough to allow us to find a faulty gene in his family, finding genes in other families with ataxia could help us to understand what was causing his lack of coordination. This in turn had the potential to point us toward an effective treatment.

In 1991, a colleague at Baylor College of Medicine, Dr. Huda Zoghbi, reported a large family in which many members had ataxia.

Using methods similar to those we later used to locate the Parkinson disease gene (Appendix 11), her genetics laboratory identified a gene for spinocerebellar ataxia (SCA) very close to genetic markers on chromosome number six.[1] Because it was the first of several SCA genes to be found, it was designated SCA1. Reports like Huda's are extremely important because they allow geneticists to determine if the same gene causes the disease in a family that they are following.

Shortly before Huda reported her findings, I had begun compiling family histories of the ataxia patients seen by our department neurologists. One family began with a twenty-eight year old named Jerry. Tall and slight of frame, with dark eyes and hair, he was devilishly handsome, but so unsteady with ataxia that I was concerned about his ability to drive himself from his home in Connecticut to our center in New Jersey. Jerry knew some of his cousins were similarly affected and, when he learned of our search for large families, he promised to trace his roots.

Jerry called me one day, exclaiming, "Alice, I've hit pay dirt!"

"Great, what is that?" I was unprepared for his answer. He'd found the family bible, traced the family back six generations, and was delighted with his discovery.

Pay dirt didn't begin to describe Jerry's find. He had identified fourteen people in his grandmother's generation, seven of whom had ataxia, and those seven had passed the disease down to some fourteen descendants. Jerry's family had been prominent in Colonial times, so I was lucky to find several published genealogies. I was able to connect this family to previous reports of families with a neurological illness, and to trace two lines of male descent back to brothers born in 1728 and 1729.

There were, of course, no medical records available from the 1700's, but that bible was the next best thing. The brothers were married to two sisters, both of whom lived well into their nineties. Had the wives had the disease, they would never have lived that long. Therefore, it had to have been the two brothers from whom subsequent generations inherited the disease. The brothers' father was born in 1688 and, surprisingly for the seventeenth century, lived to be 100 years old! Again, because no one with the disease lives to be that old, I felt certain that the disease gene had to have been introduced to the brothers by their mother.

That woman's father was known to be a French Huguenot who emigrated to North America shortly after the revocation of the Edict of Nantes (1598), and who figured prominently in the French and Indian War, but there my disease tracing ended. The brothers' surname was Whipple, so we dubbed them "the W family." If a female had interrupted the male line of descent, a name change in marriage might have precluded my being able to trace this pedigree. It is not uncommon for discoveries in science, particularly genetics, to depend on such a roll of the dice.

Ten is a magic number to a geneticist. With DNA samples from ten affected individuals, plus their unaffected relatives, we have the mathematical power to determine where a given gene maps on the chromosomes. Ten of the thirty "W" family members with ataxia were still living. They were scattered throughout the United States. Roger Duvoisin, neurology fellow Dr. Thomas Zimmerman, and I set out to visit them all. We conducted neurological examinations, made videotapes to document clinical signs, and drew blood samples in living rooms from New England to the West Coast.

We met two sisters, both suffering from ataxia, who lived in a lakeside cottage in Ohio. One sister already was severe enough to be wheelchair-bound, yet they entertained us with a resilient humor. Dr. Tom is tall, thin, bow-tied, and sufficiently young looking that he was often taken for my son. I will never forget Dr. Tom's voice as he broke into a rendition of "Indian Love Call," the sun slowly setting over that lake in Ohio. Jeanette MacDonald herself would have warmed to his ability to put our patients at ease.

We met a father of three in California whose relative had appeared in *Ripley's Believe It Or Not*, riding a horse upright through a gaping hole in a giant redwood tree. The father had mounted safety grab-bars on the walls throughout his house, so that his three adult daughters with ataxia could maneuver more safely. We even traveled to Connecticut, met Jerry's immediate family, and shared in the plans for his upcoming wedding celebration.

Once I had the "W" family blood samples safely back home, I set to work in the lab. I managed to determine that the "W" family gene was not the same SCA1 that Dr. Zoghbi had found on chromosome six. Negative studies—ruling something out—frequently do not get published. However, in the case of the "W" family, I thought that other researchers, working on branches of the same family, would appreciate being made aware of my findings and spared wasting resources repeating the same search. I published my results[2] and began the hunt for a different gene, one that would turn out to be SCA3.

In 1993 I attended a meeting on the Isle of Capri to report our findings on this family. My group photo outside the 4-star La Palma hotel includes the top fifty leaders in the field of ataxia research from throughout the world. Many wore their National Ataxia Foundation tee shirts featuring a yellow and black-checkered cab cartoon and the statement, "Ataxia is not a foreign cab."

Conspicuously absent from the Capri photograph is Anita Harding from England, an integral contributor to the research field, whose name is synonymous with ataxia research. Anita had been diagnosed with cancer in her early forties. She died not long after the Capri meeting, just before she was to take up the Chair in Clinical Neurology at the Institute of Neurology in Queen Square, London. Seeing such a life cut short changes one's perspective on the "publish-or-perish" cry that drives academia. It identifies the real urgency of what we do as scientists and reminds me, too, how breakthroughs never come quickly enough for a patient desperately waiting for a cure to his or her disease.

One of the researchers present in the picture is Jorge Sequeiros from Portugal. A tall, shy man with laughing eyes, Jorge is internationally recognized as the clinical expert in a specific type of ataxia, called Machado-Joseph disease (MJD). The name "Machado-Joseph" comes from two families of Portuguese/Azorean descent.

They were among the first families described with the disease during the 1970s.

During an afternoon free of scheduled meetings, Jorge and I climbed to Capri's peak at Anna Capri. His easy manner made me feel as if we had been long time friends. I was flattered when Jorge confided in me that he had located the gene for MJD. Scientific results are typically carefully guarded until they are published, lest they be stolen or "scooped." As we shared a boat ride to Capri's Blue Grotto, Jorge told me that he thought the clinical description of the Whipple family members was most consistent with MJD. I trusted his clinical expertise and, excitedly, planned the experiments that I was going to conduct upon returning home to our William Dow Lovett Laboratory for Neurogenetics. If he was right, I could shorten the process of finding the "W" family gene from years to a matter of weeks.

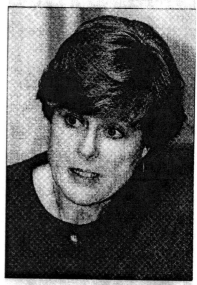

Patient's family tree yields clues to genetic ailment

Dr. Alice Lazzarini wants to map the genes of large families affected by neurological disorders

Star-Ledger February 24, 1991

I wished Jorge joy in his discovery, but within weeks after that meeting, a Japanese publication reported the location of MJD on chromosome number fourteen. Jorge was too much of a gentleman to have let it show but, after devoting his entire career to the study of one disease, he had to have been disappointed to be beaten in the race to uncover its cause. As the Portuguese were the first

Europeans to enter Japan centuries ago, the Japanese cases likely originated in Jorge's homeland.

Jorge turned out to be right about the "W" family and I finally was able to put a name to the "W" family's disease and to offer genetic counseling to family members. The third ataxia gene to be located, MJD became known as SCA3.

I believe strongly that the families that participate so generously in research deserve to be kept informed of the progress being made. However, research results cannot be release to an individual until the findings are confirmed. Test results must then be standardized in a laboratory that is certified to release information for use in medical decision-making. I developed a periodic newsletter as a way to apprise the family of potential clinical implications for themselves. By the spring of 1995, in volume III, No 1 of the "W Family Newsletter" (Appendix I), I was able to announce, "Our work and your help have paid off. We have found the 'W' family gene."

Chapter XIV
DR. BILL AND DR. ALICE

While I was coordinating the HDFSC, Mike McCormack frequently had encouraged me to finish my PhD. However, there was hardly the opportunity to do so. I was too busy working fifty or sixty-hour weeks to keep up with the HD families who were in need of assistance. Starting in 1979 with my first patient, Linda, our program had grown to include several hundred families. Taking time off to pursue a degree was simply not an option.

Roger Duvoisin not only expressed that same faith in my ability, but he also provided me with the opportunity to complete my doctorate. He knew that with an advanced degree, I could better command research monies, and survive when he retired. Much of my coursework was complete, so at that juncture I had only to do my qualifying exams and complete a research thesis. Roger was able to continue to pay my salary as long as I could intersperse my research with work in fulfillment of the ataxia endowment. I would have to work like hell, but it was the opportunity of a lifetime. He suggested that I do my research under my boss, the medical doctor whom he had hired to direct the William Dow Lovett Laboratory for Neurogenetics, Dr. William G. Johnson.

Dr. Bill's round face, pug nose and youthful appearance countered his sixty plus years. He combed a full head of poker straight reddish-blonde hair to one side where it rose to a point on the crown of his head. A matching full, blunt cut moustache graced his upper lip. Seeing him walk with his feet turned slightly outward, conjured a vision of Charlie Chaplin. In winter chill or summer heat, he wore the same herringbone, wool-tweed jacket, and its shoulder pads did little to fill in his rounded shoulders. A brilliant graduate of

Princeton, his awkward social responses frequently left people confused about their interactions with him.

Dr. Bill's reputation preceded him. While at Columbia, he had specialized in biochemical genetics, testing babies for metabolic disorders like Tay-Sachs disease. But, colleagues complained, many a new mother agonized over the fate of her newborn while waiting for results to be released from his lab. He could not let anything go without re-re-re-checking. In shifting over to the newer field of molecular genetics, he relied on a twenty-something whippersnapper lab technician whom he had brought with him from Columbia. The whipper-snapper was extremely bright, and very personable, but it didn't seem to matter that he was not very neat.

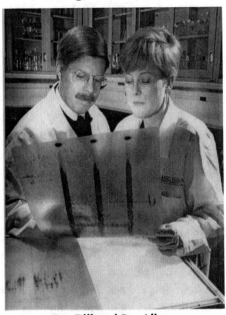

Dr. Bill and Dr. Alice

When I first entered the William Dow Lovett Laboratory for Neurogenetics I stood gawking in dismay. There was not a single, cleared, laboratory bench surface. Piles of paper were strewn in utter disarray. Used laboratory equipment lay in no particular order. Samples appeared randomly scattered on countertops.

I never had worked in a DNA laboratory, but Sr. Anna Catherine had schooled me well in the absolute need for cleanliness and precision in all laboratory work. Working with DNA, one manipulates miniscule amounts of material that, with any mishandling, could easily become contaminated with one's own DNA or with DNA from another sample. Because individual DNAs are stored and re-sampled for each separate experiment, a sample switch can lead to erroneous results for an entire series of experiments. Guarding against contamination from sloppy laboratory practices is particularly critical. I struggled to keep the DNA samples on which I was working separate and free from contamination. These included the "W" family and other ataxia samples; samples from two families with mental retardation which I was using for my research thesis; samples from families with Restless Leg syndrome upon which I collaborated with another researcher; an ever growing number of Parkinson disease samples; and assorted control samples from collaborators.

Our lab had a computerized database of information on patients' samples that I was told not to use lest I make a mistake entering information. Ironically, once I finally wheedled access to the precious database, I found so many errors that I expended much of my time just correcting them. I was new to the techniques of the molecular genetics laboratory, and like Dr. Bill, I needed the whippersnapper's expertise. I strove, therefore, to hide my disgust at the disorganization. But, when I could no longer contain myself, I went through the lab straightening up and organizing like a whirling dervish. Within a day or so, the entire lab again looked as if a nor'easter had plowed through it leaving chaos in its wake.

As my work on ataxia was in his lab, it made sense that Dr. Bill would become my PhD mentor and that he chair my committee. Most PhD research is in basic research, showing the mechanism by which a cell might use a certain protein, for instance, but the questions to which I sought answers were clinical and motivated by the needs of my patients.

I have always been an idealist and strongly identified with Cervantes's Don Quixote. Some have suggested my tendency to crusade is closer to Joan of Arc. Indeed, you may agree when I tell you that I set out to prove my mentor wrong—the very same mentor who headed the committee that would grant my degree.

As a neurologist Dr. Bill had diagnosed a boy with a specific form of sex-linked mental retardation (inherited by males and passed through the females just like Prince Alexei's hemophilia). I found a publication of a newly described sex-linked retardation that seemed to better fit the patient's symptoms—one that I could prove in the laboratory. I also included in my research thesis another family with sex-linked mental retardation whom I had counseled. I knew that if I could find the location of the genes in these two families, I could identify female carriers and provide them with genetic counseling. This became my very clinically oriented research project.

Writing my thesis was a grueling process. Each time that Dr. Bill was able to find small edits, he took out his inch-thick, phallic-looking pen. I'd see that pen whip out of the breast pocket of that wool-tweed coat and my stomach would tighten into knots. I knew I would be spending the following night at the computer making the requested alterations. The next day we'd go over the exact same material and there would be different iterations. I tried to assume a Machiavellian approach, telling myself that the end justified the means—I will finish my PhD! I just hoped it wouldn't be posthumously!

By the time my oral defense was scheduled, my thesis no longer seemed to be written in English, but some foreign tongue that I could not decipher. Nevertheless, I had swallowed my need for a clean workspace; I had spent endless hours in the lab running gel after DNA gel and analyzing results; I had suffered the phallic pen's invasion—nothing was going to stand in the way of my finally earning my PhD at fifty-six years of age.

My family and a dear friend attended my oral thesis presentation for moral support, as did the whippersnapper. Stage fright prevailed, but I got through my presentation. I fielded questions from the five-member committee regarding my methodology and conclusions. I was feeling almost victorious when one of the committee members said somberly, "Alice, would you and your guests please leave the room while we discuss your work."

As I waited outside in the dark hallway everything felt surreal, a clock ticking in slow motion. I had done all I could do. Their verdict was now beyond my ability to control.

My supporters tried to bolster me. "Mom, you did an awesome job," said Rob.

"I'm so proud of you," said Kathi.

"I couldn't understand a word of it, but it sounded great," said my friend.

Finally Dr. Bill came to get me. The mood was solemn. Suddenly I did not feel so victorious.

Several members of my committee were skeptical that my research constituted a valid enough project to merit a PhD, but it was Dr. Bill who defended my work to the committee and argued for my being granted the degree. As each member affixed a signature to my thesis face page, bearing witness that I had passed, it didn't matter that they weren't ebullient over my work, that the mood in the room was reluctance. What mattered was that I had persisted in following my dream. With Dr. Bill standing in my corner, I had prevailed. And in the end, he was not at all threatened, but seemed appreciative to have a correct diagnosis for his patient. His gracious generosity made me forget all the aggravation I had endured in the process...almost.

In May of 1996 my entire family was present at the graduation ceremony as I received my PhD in Cell and Developmental Biology jointly from Rutgers University and the University of Medicine and Dentistry of New Jersey.

Kathi had gotten her MD in 1990. So as not to be confused with her physician father-in-law, she retained her maiden name. I asked her, "How do you feel about my also being 'Dr. Lazzarini,' even though I'm not a 'real' doctor like you?"

"Don't worry about them confusing us, Mom, and you're every bit as real a doctor as I am," she replied with genuine pride in her voice.

Chapter XV
THE BOSS AND PARKINSON DISEASE

"I want to work on stroke," Roger Duvoisin had declared when Houston Merritt hired him.

"But I need you to take over the Parkinson's clinic," Merritt had countered.

Roger was allowed to continue his work on stroke—but only as long as he also ran the Parkinson's program. As the first fellow of the Parkinson Disease Foundation, he ran Columbia Presbyterian's Parkinson's Clinic in New York City from 1962 to 1973. Similarly, I staked my ground in making the transition to Roger's department. "I prefer my fun loving Huntington patients to those stiff 'Parkies,'" I insisted. To me, the dance-like movements that one sees in Huntington patients represent a wonderfully free loss of inhibition and spontaneous behavior. The cautious rigidity seen in Parkinson's patients screamed, BORING. But few people were able to work for the Boss without getting pulled into working on Parkinson disease (PD).

Shortly after I transitioned to full time in his department, Roger said, "Alice, I want you to prove Parkinson's is genetic."

I gulped, took a deep breath, and immediately began to think through how I might go about satisfying his tall order. I had no way of knowing to what degree I would become part of his far-reaching legacy. Nor could I have foreseen how the entire world of Parkinson's research would make a 180-degree turn because of one man's vision, courage, and salmon-like tenacity, in swimming against the current of a deeply entrenched idea.

Since James Parkinson described the "shaking palsy" in 1817, neurologists had put forth different theories about the cause of Parkinson disease, from environmental exposure, to infectious disease, to inheritance. "Boss" Houston Merritt had held to the idea that Parkinson's was a syndrome of varied causes, and "Boss" Roger Duvoisin, Merritt's protégé and title heir, spent his career trying to define its fundamental nature.

During the early 1960's, Dr. David Poskanzer at Harvard was arguing that PD was viral—a result of the epidemic of encephalitis—and that it would disappear by 1980. Unconvinced, Roger painstakingly reviewed patient records at the Massachusetts General Hospital and showed Poskanzer's analysis had been faulty. Roger reasoned that if PD were caused by an isolated epidemic, the number of PD cases would peak following that epidemic. When he moved to Presbyterian Hospital, he reviewed all the medical records of Parkinson's patients seen there from 1880 through 1962, and he found no change in the number of PD cases over the eighty-two-year span.

Then, working in Presbyterian's newly established Parkinson's Brain Bank, Roger collaborated with neuropathology fellow Manuel Stadlan. Roger identified traits that had been found in clinical examination while Manny examined the corresponding pathology. Only after they were finished did they compare their findings: individuals who had had encephalitis showed a distinct pathology from that which came to be known as "Lewy-body Parkinson disease," further solidifying Roger's conviction.

At Columbia, Roger was instrumental in designing what became the Hoehn-Yahr scale, a tool that is still relied on for determining the stages of Parkinson disease. He was also part of the L-dopa treatment breakthrough, so poignantly depicted by Robert De Niro's performance as a man with parkinsonism in the movie, *Awakenings*. *L-dopa*, marketed initially as *Sinemet*, is now sold as the generic, *carbidopa/levodopa*, but it remains the standard of care for the treatment of Parkinson disease.

In *Awakenings*, Robin Williams portrayed De Niro's pioneering neurologist, who successfully used this new medication to "awaken" his catatonic patients. In the movie, De Niro's character had the form of parkinsonism that occurs as a result of a brain infection, and once medication was stopped, he and the other patients quickly reverted to their stupefied state. Thankfully, the drug's effectiveness is longer lasting for Parkinson disease.

Initially, Roger was convinced that PD was not genetic. An astute clinician, without formal training in genetics, he intuited the importance of comparing identical with non-identical twins, and began to collect twin pairs from his PD clinic. Pairs of identical twins share all the same genes whereas fraternal twins, like any two siblings, share only half their genes. Because Roger found the same number of like cases in both identical and fraternal twin pairs, he argued vehemently to his colleagues against a genetic contribution to PD.

In 1973 Roger had left Columbia for a sabbatical at King's College Hospital in London, after which he joined Mt. Sinai School of Medicine back in New York City. In 1979, he became Chairman of Neurology at Robert Wood Johnson (RWJ) Medical School where he continued to observe more familial cases of PD. He decided to comb through his twin-study data. When one of his identical twins developed PD long after his co-twin, Roger wondered, could his data have been misleading? Was there really an underlying genetic component to PD?

Then, in 1986 a patient enrolled in an experimental drug trial at RWJ. The patient was doing well, but suffered an unrelated accidental death. Roger had seen a member of the same family in the 1960's and recorded a bit of positive family history, so he prevailed on the medical examiner to release the brain to his neuropathologist. When the pathology showed Lewy bodies, the hallmark of Parkinson disease, Roger knew he had found the first-ever, autopsy-proven case of inherited PD.

Immediately after the funeral, the patient's brother contacted Dr. Larry Golbe for treatment of his own Parkinson's. Then another trial participant with PD turned out to be a distant cousin of the two brothers. As the family originated from Contursi, Italy, a village of 5,000 some sixty-five miles southeast of Naples, Roger contacted the chair of Neurology at the *Seconda Universita degli Studi di Napoli* who put him in touch with Dr. Giuseppe Di Iorio. Giuseppe agreed to collaborate to identify family members in Italy, examine them and draw blood samples. Most family members welcomed Giuseppe and were willing to contribute a blood sample, but at one Italian farmhouse Giuseppe found himself looking down the barrel of a shotgun. He wisely decided to forgo collecting that sample.

Once Larry tracked down extended families in the United States and family members who had emigrated from Contursi to Argentina, Germany, and northern Italy, 400 family members were identified that spanned twelve generations. Sixty-one of the 400 descendants of a couple who lived in Contursi in the late seventeenth century were found to have, or have had, PD. I had studied a number of other families in which multiple persons were affected with Parkinson disease. But, a family in which the disease affected generation after generation, and in which there were at least ten samples available from affected individuals, was a geneticist's dream; It gives us the mathematical power to identify the disease-causing gene, the promise of understanding how a disease develops, and the potential to generate more effective treatments.

Larry recognized the importance of making the scientific community aware of this family's existence. He published the first paper on the "Contursi" kindred, the largest known multi-case Parkinson's family in the world.[1] This began a scientific journey that would change the future of Parkinson's research.

At the International PD Symposium in Jerusalem circa 1990, Larry presented the pathology for the Contursi family member who had died. This made a huge scientific stir, as it was the first time anyone had reported typical PD pathology in a familial case, and thus established credence for a genetic cause. At that meeting Roger stood up and announced that he had changed his mind and that he now believed that PD had a genetic component. Roger would later tell me that, "Some people were especially vituperative in denouncing my new view. I had a tiger by the tail and clearly needed a clinical geneticist to collect and analyze genealogies and study the patterns of inheritance. Hence I hired you!"

Just as Roger had combed through patients' medical records at Massachusetts General Hospital and then at Presbyterian Hospital, so I spent long hours combing through hundreds of charts from his Parkinson's patients, contacting family members, and documenting whether there were any additional affected relatives. I called on a long-time friend from my days working with Huntington's, Dr. Rick Myers at Boston University School of Medicine, to help with the analysis. In 1994, he and my colleagues at Robert Wood Johnson Medical School co-authored my paper in the journal, *Neurology*, supporting a genetic underpinning to PD.[2]

Given that Parkinson disease typically begins about sixty-three years of age, many persons with Parkinson disease are unable to provide complete medical histories for their parents. In compiling family histories on over 200 Parkinson's patients, we showed that once that lack of medical information on these first-degree relatives was taken into account, the evidence for Parkinson disease having a genetic component became stronger. When I reported these findings at the American Academy of Neurology meeting, it helped to turn the tide of thinking about the cause of PD.

Between his reanalysis of the twin data, the response to my paper, and finding the Contursi kindred, Roger Duvoisin had become the neurology community's strongest proponent for a genetic cause of PD.

Listening to a 2010 webcast panel discussion of the drug-development pipeline, I heard one audience member ask about the effect of a paradigm shift when someone realizes that an accepted theory fundamentally changes. He wanted to know what happens to drug development when an idea that researchers had been wedded to by virtue of long research careers and funding history is turned upside down. Dr. Story Landis, director of NINDS, answered by citing Roger's shift in thought from espousing an environmental cause of PD to accommodating a role for genetics. Dr. Landis explained how it brought about a change in PD research from the bench of the basic scientist to the way we approach potential therapeutics. Thus, more than twenty years later, the importance of Roger's willingness to pioneer such a paradigm shift is still lauded.

༈

In August 1995, Roger had attended a workshop on Parkinson disease sponsored by the National Institutes of Health (NIH). He had with him a copy of the pedigree of the Contursi family, which he called to the attention of Dr. Robert Nussbaum, Chief of the Laboratory of Genetic Diseases at NIH's National Human Genome Research Institute. Nussbaum was impressed both with my analysis of PD families and with the Contursi pedigree. Dr. Zachary Hall, then Director of the National Institute of Neurological Disorders and Stroke (NINDS), phoned Roger at home to propose collaborating to accelerate the search for the Contursi-family gene.

Roger accepted Dr. Hall's offer of collaboration. The Contursi samples were to be sent to the laboratory of Dr. Nussbaum's colleague at NIH, Mihaelis Polymeropoulos. NIH, in turn, provided funding toward my salary so that I might oversee the sharing of samples from our laboratory and collect any additional samples that were needed.

In order to find the gene, we needed to have blood samples from family members, both affected and unaffected. Some of the Contursi samples had been collected and were already stored in our laboratory in New Jersey. I undertook a campaign to collect the remaining samples and, for the next year, I was in daily communication with the laboratory.

Then, in September 1996, Mihaelis phoned me, saying, "Alice, we've got results. How fast could you go to Contursi to collect some additional samples?" That was Contursi, ITALY. But I didn't speak Italian! He went on, "I'm sure we have a hit, but one woman's sample shows conflicting results. I need you to go to Contursi ASAP and collect additional samples."

The lab had been working on mapping another disease and, coincidentally, happened to be using markers for chromosome 4. When these markers were tested against the Contursi samples, our gene quickly revealed its hiding place on chromosome 4.

"I'll need a few days to make arrangements and get my passport renewed," I told him, struggling to contain the implications of his news: in just a matter of months, he had found the location of the faulty Contursi-family gene, and I was to be an ambassador of NIH!

My son, thirty-one-years-old at the time, had spent a year studying art in Florence, so I arranged for him to accompany me as translator. In a flurry of activity, I bought tickets, got an expedited passport renewal, packed, and we were Italy bound within four days.

Chapter XVI
CONTURSI

September 1996.

Just eight weeks earlier, TWA Flight 800 flying from JFK to France had exploded at 13,000 feet and crashed into the Atlantic Ocean off East Moriches, Long Island, killing all 230 persons on board. Rumors circulate that it was shot down by a missile.

We are flying out of JFK. We are on TWA. It is Friday the 13th. As we taxi onto the runway, I work at keeping myself focused on the job at hand. I am the National Institutes of Health's overseas emissary for a team on the brink of reporting the first gene to cause Parkinson disease, a disease that devastates the lives of millions of people worldwide.

"Mom," Rob brings me out of my reverie. "The plane has stopped taxiing. They're cranking up some sort of crane with lots of equipment. I think there's something wrong with the engine."

"Well, I'm sure the airline won't let the pilot take this sucker across the big pond if anything is wrong with it." I try to reassure him—and myself.

Rob sees his chance to toy with my nervousness a bit. "Mom, it's better they find something that needs fixing now than while we're out over the ocean. But, if we should go down, I can't think of anyone I'd rather crash into the Atlantic Ocean with than you."

"I'm glad, dear. I feel the same way...I guess."

We are delayed an hour while they fix what I don't want to know might be broken. Finally we are airborne. I go back to thinking about my good fortune: a career that allows me to travel to exotic places and work on the cutting edge of a field that I love.

"Mom," comes Rob's voice again. "I can see the lights of East Moriches below us. I think I see debris floating in the water."

"The pilot certainly doesn't want to crash. He's not going to fly something that's not in ship shape."

But, might there *really be someone out there firing missiles at airplanes?* I keep my concern to myself, choosing not to give Rob more fodder for banter.

We land in Rome, and after a night's sleep, have a single day to play tourist. Rob has been here before. I have not. St. Peter's square, the piazza San Pietro, is a must see. Given our last minute preparations, I had not had time to contact a priest-friend who works in the Vatican to inquire how one gets an audience with Pope.

I wake Rob early, my voice now the insistent one. "Rob, rise and shine."

"Let me sleep just a bit longer. I was out late last night."

"We have one day to see the entire city, and you're not going to spend it in bed," I cajol, tossing off his covers.

Rob rises, showers away the fuzzy night before, and off we go on our adventure.

We head to the Vatican. Observing that somber fortress, I felt as if it had been there forever. I have been to other parts of Europe, and appreciate the flavor of old, a flavor that one cannot begin to taste in the States, but the Vatican is *really* old.

"At noon on Sundays Pope John Paul II gives a blessing from his window in the Apostolic Palace, the second from the right on the top floor," says the guidebook.

"It's Sunday. The Pope is waiting for me," I inform my personal translator and guide. I assume that since Pope John Paul II has Parkinson's disease, and I am in Italy on an important Parkinson's research mission, that fate has brought us together. As we approach the *Piazza San Pietro*, it seems rather strange that there are no people. A small phalanx of black-clad nuns, and plenty of pigeons, but no crowds and no Pope!

"Where do you suppose everyone is?" I ask Rob.

"Perhaps the Pope heard you were coming and skipped town."

In time we learn the Pope had done just that, having switched to his winter schedule. Stood up by the Pope!

The next day we take the train to Naples where our colleague Dr. Giuseppe Di Iorio meets us at the station. Forty-one-year-old Giuseppe is formally dressed in a suit and tie. Slight, olive-skinned with chiseled Roman features, Giuseppe has an unassuming demeanor. He and *Roberto* become fast friends and thoroughly enjoy their futile attempt to get me to pronounce *grazie* with some modicum of an Italian accent. Although unable to understand their banter, I suspect what I am witnessing is two charming Italian men, each out-charming the other.

We speed south along Italy's Amalfi coast in Guiseppe's silver Alfa Romeo. Spectacular new panoramas appear with each bend in the road. Looking out over the green Mediterranean Sea, I surrender to the sun's warmth and the sweet smell of citrus blossoms wafting through the open window. We stop for lunch at the Zaccaria restaurant, a fresh-from-the-sea repast, replete with Limoncello, the local lemon-based liquor. (It does help to quell the queasiness of that perilous ride.) The Duomo of Amalfi surprises us with its oriental-style mosaic facade.

"Saint Andrew's bones are interred under the altar," Giuseppe tells us. "Amalfi was a maritime republic that rivaled Venice. Its trade routes extended as far as Constantinople, where the bronze doors of the Duomo were forged in 1066." Pointing with pride, he adds, "That bronze statue in the piazza near the harbor is Flavio Gioia inventor of the compass."

Dusk finds us on the high cliffs above Amalfi in the Villa Rufolo gardens. Giuseppe tells us "Richard Wagner orchestrated his opera, Parsifal here. When he came upon these gardens he exclaimed, 'the magic garden of Klingsor has been found.'"

How poetic to be standing here in Wagner's magic garden on the threshold of a grand discovery.

Finally, navigating by moonlight, we find the tiny Contursi hotel precariously perched on the side of a mountain. After settling in, we locate an empty conference room off the lobby where Giuseppe and I unroll a scroll containing our subject's family's history onto a large table. Geneticists call such a medical history a "pedigree," and this large account is twenty pages in length. Before meeting family members, we need to review the clinical details for accuracy and make sure that we agree on some key relationships. Giuseppe (in Italian) and I (in English) depend on our artist's translation.

"Are we sure this woman here on page two is the second cousin, once removed, to this man on page fourteen?" I ask.

"Mom, what's a second cousin once removed?" queries Rob.

"It's the relationship of a child of one second cousin to the other second cousin. Here, let me draw you a picture."

"Now you're talking my language." He translates my question into Italian.

"Did this man have his onset at twenty or twenty-five?" I ask, pointing to a small square on the diagram.

"Do you mean onset of symptoms, or when he was diagnosed?" Rob's question comes back.

"His age when the symptoms started."

"Twenty-five," he answers.

Pointing to a square labeled IV-25[1], I ask, "How do we get autopsy tissue on this man?"

"God, Mom, that's really gross," Rob responds.

"Please, can you just translate so we can finish this?"

"It should be at the hospital in Naples," Rob relays. "Are we done yet?"

We review the pedigree well into night, stopping only for a few cappuccinos.

The next morning, our first patient meets us at our hotel. Like Rob, he is in his early thirties. Parkinson disease in the Contursi kindred is similar to ordinary Parkinson's, except that it occurs at an earlier age. Our patient shuffles toward us. Stooped slightly, he looks up as we greet him, his face devoid of expression.

"My God," Rob utters as he absorbs the reality of his peer's predicament. Our Italian patient struggles to walk across the patio that lies between them. Rob has his entire life in front of him. Our young man has maybe ten years remaining, and they are already arduous ones. He will likely soon be debilitated to the point of being unable to walk, talk or even smile as Parkinson's steals his ability to move. That single moment in time etches itself into my memory and into my heart. My son's introduction to Parkinson disease is a poignant one.

After examining and obtaining a blood sample from our first patient, we drive to the center of the small village and meet our other collaborator, local general practitioner Dr. Salvatore La Sala. Salvatore is a rotund, middle-aged, white-haired gentleman whose demeanor inspires the same trust as would Norman Rockwell's general practitioner. Salvatore is himself a member of the Contursi kindred, but is unaffected. Salvatore has arranged for the family members to come to his office. They understand that we "outsiders" are there to try to help solve the mystery of their family's disease. Salvatore draws blood from seven family members. Then he hits trouble.

A woman cloaked in heavy, dark garb comes into the office with her son. Her age is known only by reference to our pedigree. This woman's blood is critical for our study in order to resolve some conflicting laboratory results. When we trace a gene through a family, we need to have samples from unaffected individuals, as well as from people who marry into the family, to compare against samples from the individuals who are affected. The son gives a sample of his blood but, when it comes time to draw the mother's, she objects.

"No, no," she shakes her head and waves her hands from side to side in front of Salvatore's face.

I want to coax, "Your blood sample is the most important of all. If we don't have your blood we may never get the definitive answer as to what is causing this devastating illness in your family." But, I don't speak her language. I can do nothing but witness the commotion.

I seek Rob's attention for a translation. "What is her difficulty?" I plead.

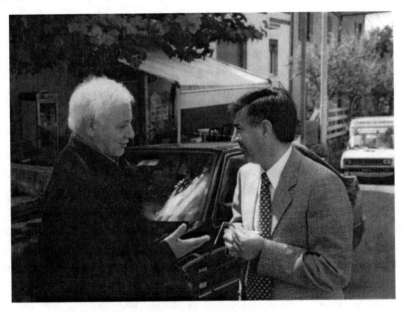

Salvatore and Giuseppe

He waves at me to wait.

How can I wait? I contemplate how I will explain to the National Institutes of Health that, having spent thousands of taxpayer's dollars, I failed to accomplish my task. Our patient continues to object, shouting and motioning even more excitedly with her hands. Salvatore then takes her hand in his and speaks to her gently. Soon she is lying down, Salvatore has the needle in her arm, and that glorious red liquid seeps into the syringe. "She is afraid of needles," is the only explanation I receive from my triumphant colleagues as the hectic scene settles and the woman accepts accolades for her bravery. Her three vials of blood hold profound implications for millions of Parkinson patients worldwide.

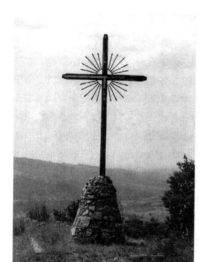

Contursi Mountain Top Cross

In a small village, the local doctor doubles as dentist and barber and is on a first name basis with everyone. As Salvatore walks us from his office down the narrow cobblestone street, women greet us hanging out of open windows and peering from street-side markets. Excited school children shout, "Dottore, Dottore." I tell Giuseppe that I would like to find a hand-painted plate with a view of Contursi as a souvenir from our trip. When we're unable to find one, he buys me a watercolor of the village painted by a local artist.

Before we leave, Salvatore drives us to the highest elevation overlooking the village. At the peak there towers a cross more than thirty feet high. "This is the final destination for religious pilgrimages by the villagers," he tells us. There are no pilgrimages this day, but it is no less a spiritual experience to be atop that mountain with my son, two wonderful new colleagues, and eight carefully packed samples that will contribute to understanding one of the world's most devastating disorders.

As we leave to head back to Naples, I realize that I had taken many close-up photographs, but I did not have a panorama with which to remember the quaint village. I hand Rob my camera and ask that he photograph a long shot from the car. Giuseppe pulls off the road, barely, and Rob takes a quick snapshot.

Back home, our precious cargo safely delivered to the lab, my teenage nephew inadvertently opens my camera. *Long shot ruined!* But, upon processing my photos I am surprised to find the panorama only partially exposed. Much of it remains salvageable.

Once the Italian samples confirm our findings, my research team plans to submit the results for publication in *Science*. Even as I traveled, my colleagues had been writing the paper. I take the salvaged Contursi panorama to my medical school's audio-visual department. They mock-up a *Science* cover by superimposing the Contursi kindred pedigree upon the partially sun streaked photo. Once *Science* accepts our paper, I offer our mock-up to the editors, but we decided not to wait in line for a spot on the cover.

Science publishes our paper in its November 15th issue.[2] The cover features someone else's research, but inside my twelve coauthors and I break major news that appears in *The New York Times*. The headline trumpets news that gives hope to millions of Parkinson disease patients worldwide: "Scientists Identify Site of Gene Tied to Some Cases of Parkinson's."

My framed *Science* cover mock-up hangs in my office next to my watercolor of Contursi Terme, a stylized interpretation of the little hillside village. Sunrays illuminate a tiny cluster of ancient buildings, and I can feel again the warmth of a time when the paths of colleagues, friends and pioneering science so intimately crossed my own.

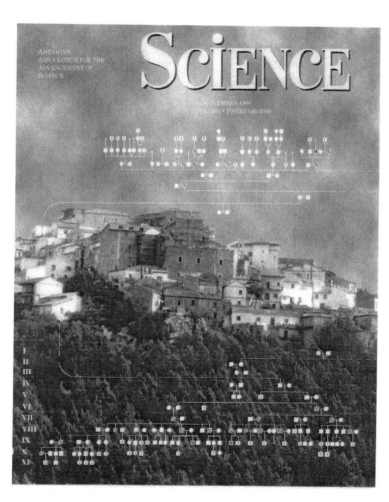

Science cover mock-up

Chapter XVII
DISCOVERY OF PARK1

November 1996, Washington DC

Larry Golbe and I find seats in the first row at the National Press Club. News cameras line the entire back windowed wall: CBS, ABC, local stations with letters I don't recognize. A poster-size diagram stands on an easel behind the podium. It boasts the location of the first Parkinson disease gene on chromosome 4—our gene! Flanking tables draped in a gold-colored cloth hold placards with the names of each person who would speak at the press conference: Dr. Harold Varmus, the Director of NIH, Dr. Zachary Hall, Director of the National Institute of Neurological Disorders and Stroke, Dr. Nussbaum, Chief of Genetic Diseases at NIH's National Human Genome Research Institute, Dr. Mihaelis Polymeropoulos and Dr. Roger Duvoisin.

I am thrilled for Roger. His career is winding down, he is getting pressure to retire, and it is glorious to see him reap such reward after a long and productive career devoted to Parkinson disease. At the moment I take his photograph, Roger is standing on Mount Everest, pointer in hand, indicating where his victory flag should rest.

I am thrilled, as well, when our breakthrough makes *The New York Times* that day. Back in New Jersey, *The Star Ledger* features our breakthrough on the front page. Other newspapers and our medical school publicity department clamor for coverage of our success. "Local team makes good" makes for wonderful news.

Finding the location of any gene is exciting, but it is just the first step in identifying that gene. Once the Huntington's gene was located in 1983, I lived through the ten-year search for the gene to be identified. I had shared the frustration of researchers laboriously inching toward their goal. I had participated in predictive testing in which the life-altering results had as high as a five percent chance of

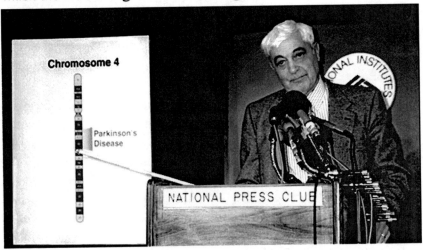

Dr. Duvoisin at The National Press Club

being wrong. But technology had advanced, and our gene was more forthcoming than the HD gene had been. Even as Rob and I traveled to Contursi, Mihaelis was at work on its identity. He had searched multiple databases seeking any gene that mapped close to the same area on chromosome 4 and also functioned in the brain. The gene that encodes *alpha-synuclein* proved to be just such a candidate. Mihaelis quickly examined DNA samples from the family members to look for a specific change in the DNA, or "mutation," within the *alpha-synuclein* gene. To be causative, each individual in the family who was affected had to have that same mutation.

Bingo!

Just seven months after publishing the paper that localized the gene on chromosome 4, we reported the specific mutation that caused PD in the Contursi kindred.[1] The initial gene localization had been in large part the luck of having had chromosome 4 markers on the laboratory bench, but this time fortune shone on the prepared mind. The affected individuals all had a mutation in the gene coding for the *alpha-synuclein* protein. As specific mutations are often named according to the disease they cause, it was called PARK1.

$\maltese$

Once the excitement had died down and the press that had inundated our laboratory packed up their cable-video cameras, I set about looking for the same mutation in blood samples that we had in our laboratory from other Parkinson's patients of Italian descent. I found none, which suggested that the Contursi mutation was unique to one family. Soon, the same mutation was found in families in central and southwestern Greece. As the Greeks are known to have fled to southern Italy after the Ottoman Turks captured Constantinople in 1453, the mutation is likely to have been brought to southern Italy by a Greek ancestor.

Despite intense worldwide scrutiny of PD pedigrees, only a few reports of other mutations in *alpha-synuclein* exist: in 1998, a mutation which causes a slightly different pattern of disease was described in a large German family, and in 2004, a third mutation in a Spanish family was reported. An American family (known as "the Iowa kindred") was reported in which affected persons have three copies of the *alpha-synuclein* gene (designated PARK4). The disease in this family is much more severe, which tells us that the more this gene is actively producing protein the worse the disease. We call this a "gene dose-effect," and can recreate it in animal models as well.

Amazingly, a humble fruit-fly can be made to resemble human Parkinson's. When the gene equivalent to *alpha-synuclein* in the fly is manipulated so as to produce excess protein, the flies show progressive symptoms as well as brain changes that resemble human PD. When mice are made to express the mutation that we described in the Contursi kindred, they, too, show PD-like neurodegeneration and motor dysfunction leading to premature death. Such animal models are invaluable tools with which to screen the effectiveness of potential therapeutics.

The Star-Ledger

FRIDAY, NOVEMBER 15, 1996   THE NEWSPAPER FOR NEW JERSEY   35 CENTS

Unlocking secrets of Parkinson's

By Kitta MacPherson
STAR-LEDGER STAFF

From a hospital room in New Brunswick to a medieval mountaintop village in Italy, a 10-year global odyssey to track down the far-flung members of a family afflicted with a dreaded disease has proved fruitful beyond measure.

In a modern-day detective story, where gene-sleuthing proved as pivotal as gumshoe tactics, a team of scientists used blood samples collected during their journey to identify their suspect — a gene mutation responsible for Parkinson's disease.

By pinpointing the specific region in human genetic material where the flawed instructions may reside, the scientists say they have shown the existence of a strong genetic component to the disease and brought the world that much closer to a cure.

"It's absolutely exhilarating," said Dr. Lawrence Golbe, a neurologist from the University of Medicine and Dentistry of New Jersey and one of the leaders of the research team that made the discovery.

The work is described in a paper to be published today in the journal Science, written by four researchers of UMDNJ in collaboration with scientists from the National Institutes of Health and the Instituto de Scienze Neurologiche in Naples, Italy.

But the report's dry depiction of chromosomal linkages hardly conveys the human drama that led physicians from a random comment by a patient visiting the Robert Wood Johnson Medical School in New Brunswick to the rolling hills of southern Italy.

It was there, in the village of Contursi outside Naples, that researchers using clues pried from dusty records in a church sacristy found the roots of a family that has been predisposed to Parkinson's disease since the 1600s.

Parkinson's disease, first medically categorized in 1817 by the English physician James Parkinson as the "shaking palsy," is a chronic progressive disorder of late adult life characterized by tremors of the hands, muscular rigidity, slowness of movement, a stooped posture and shuffling gait.

Caused by the degeneration of nerve cells in the brain, it affects about 500,000 people in the U.S.

Attorney General Janet Reno suffers from it.

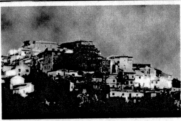

The Italian village of Contursi became the center of attention as the research team delved into a family's roots.

Many others, including the retired boxer Muhammad Ali, have Parkinson's-like symptoms due to head injury, toxic chemicals or other problems.

Scientists for decades had long suspected that there was a genetic component to the disease.

Then, about 20 years ago, they were convinced otherwise by Dr. Roger Duvoisin, the dean of Parkinson's research at UMDNJ who is an emeritus professor of neurology at UMDNJ and an author of the new research paper.

Twin studies he conducted convinced him that heredity did not play a significant role.

Chance pattern

But the prospect of a genetic link continued to haunt him, especially after he began to notice an increasing number of cases within families.

In 1986, Duvoisin and Golbe began to study the question more closely.

A chance pattern emerged early that year, when one patient mentioned his family had emigrated from Contursi and another patient phoned in about a medication problem. Golbe, thumbing through the latter patient's records, noted her family tree had a branch in Contursi.

"I believed it had to be far more than a coincidence," said Golbe, who immediately recruited a genetics expert and physician in Italy, Giuseppe Di Iorio, to help in the cause

Di Iorio, meeting with a local Roman Catholic priest in the 5,000-resident Italian hilltop village, convinced him to open up the parish files, including all births, deaths and marriages going back centuries. In this manner, the patients' genealogy could be traced.

Di Iorio found that it threaded back to one couple who came to the village in the late 1600s.

By studying genetic material and interviewing family members, the scientists were able to later conclude that the couple did not show signs of Parkinson's, but carried the gene for the disorder.

The disease did not manifest itself in family members until the early 1800s.

The gene mutation in this family is inherited in dominant fashion, meaning that people who possess the mutation have a 50 percent chance of passing it on to their children.

Searching for family

Once the familial relationship had been established, the genetic search kicked in.

Duvoisin, Golbe and Di Iorio had to track down as many living members of the family as they could find to draw blood to look for common genetic traits.

Some had migrated to the U.S. between 1890 and 1920 to cities in New Jersey, California and Florida.

Others had spread around the globe, to Germany and Argentina.

When it came to visiting strangers' homes to ask for blood, researchers ran into resistance. Alice Lazzarini, a geneticist who joined the research team in 1990 and is also an author of the research paper, has done her share of pounding the pavement.

Accompanying Di Iorio on a visit to an 80-year-old member of the family living in Contursi, she witnessed what seemed to be a vicious argument, carried out in Italian with hand gestures aplenty, between the woman and the physician.

In the end, the woman allowed the visitors to take a blood sample.

"She was afraid of needles," Lazzarini said, explaining the argument.

In another less successful case, Golbe visited a Jersey City member of the extended family three times over the past several years in an attempt to get a specimen.

October, 1998

Despite the wafting aroma of coffee, I am too excited to stop for a cup. I hurry into the dimly lit auditorium, and stand at the back letting myself savor the moment. The room is full of researchers anxiously crammed into a space intended for a much smaller group. Out-of-body-like, my head feels as though it is soaring with importance, high above the crowd.

These internationally renowned professionals are discussing the breakthroughs resulting from my team's research!

As each slide is projected onto the screen, rays of light pour forth new data. Voices buzz excitedly after each presentation as attendees discuss their implications for research. Our discovery of the mutation in *alpha-synuclein*, PARK1, has already begun to revolutionize the field of Parkinson disease research.

And, I helped to make this wonderful story happen...

The number of times and the persistence with which a paper is cited by other researchers is considered by the scientific community to be the measure of a paper's influence. My team's two *Science* papers, identifying the Contursi gene location, and then the mutation in *alpha*-synuclein, have been cited hundreds of times. A web search for "*alpha-synuclein* and Parkinson disease" will generate thousands of hits.

Further support for the importance of the discovery followed immediately upon our publication, when pathologists reported that the *alpha-synuclein* protein aggregated in Parkinson's brains.[2] One of those pathologists, a University of Pennsylvania School of Medicine professor, John Trojanowski, was quoted as saying the discovery of PARK1 had "blown open the lid on Parkinson disease."

Researchers all over the world have followed our lead, and huge amounts of resources have poured into following the path that was illuminated by our discovery. The Michael J. Fox Foundation for Parkinson's Research, one of the world's largest private sources of research monies for Parkinson disease, has funded in excess of $47 million in projects to address how *alpha-synuclein* triggers cell death, and how it might be countered so as to develop an effective treatment.

Studies of flies and mice further demonstrate that neurodegenerative pathology is reversible. This is an exciting new concept for the field of neurology, one on which Christopher Reeve expended much energy in his efforts to fund research for spinal-cord injury. Since our discovery of the *alpha-synuclein* mutation, hopes are high that we will be able to further clarify the mechanism by which disease occurs and determine how we might interrupt, perhaps reverse, the process to bring about a successful treatment. As one researcher put it, the next generation of PD treatments no doubt will be based on research that would not have been possible without the identification of that first rare mutation in *alpha-synuclein* (see Appendix II).

Chapter XVIII
FROM ACADEMIA TO INDUSTRY:
A CAREER IN PERIL

By 1996 Roger was nearing 70 years of age, and had decided it was time to retire. He had foreseen the day that he would step down, and had tried to prepare me by enabling me to finish my doctorate. The new department chairman had not been steeped in the department's tradition with Parkinson disease and other movement disorders, and he brought different priorities. He brought, as well, a determination that each faculty member would support his or her own salary. Clinicians do that by teaching and seeing patients; researchers do it by getting grants. Being dependent on the vagaries of funding priorities is referred to as being on "soft money."

In terms of soft money, my future suddenly was looking tenuous. The American Parkinson Disease Association had funded two of my grants, and I had an NIH grant pending, but as a new PhD the chances of my getting NIH funding were slim. My glib comment during my interview with Roger, "I can get along with anyone," came back to haunt me as I progressed from feeling cocky, to timid, to fearing for my job.

For a few years, Larry Golbe and other colleagues found funding in order to cobble together my salary. In 1999 I was helping Larry with research on Progressive Supranuclear Palsy (PSP), a disease with PD-like symptoms. He sent me to a conference held by his fellow PSP researchers, and I was surprised to see Mihaelis Polymeropoulos there. I had heard that he recently moved to Novartis Pharmaceuticals. It was the first time I had seen him since we published the 1997 paper on *alpha-synuclein*. Maneuvering

135

toward him through the crowd that hovered around a pastry-laden refreshment table, I grabbed a black coffee and asked Mihaelis, "How do you like industry?"

"Alice, it's very exciting, the work we're doing."

"Tell me more about what it is."

Small and boyish looking, Mihaelis was not yet forty but already had impressive research successes to his credit. Novartis had offered him a vice presidency with a package of considerable resources for him to develop the new field of pharmacogenetics. Pharmacogenetics aims to save time, money and lives by determining how an individual's genetic makeup will affect response to a given drug. It also promises to enrich the coffers of companies that can harness its potential.

"The company is investing in pharmacogenetics big time. They know that eventually all drugs will be tailored to an individual's genetic makeup," Mihaelis said.

"How exciting to be in on the ground floor of a brand new area of medicine," I told him.

"I'm keeping my lab in Maryland, but we'll have a group coordinating the clinical trials in New Jersey. Do you want to come work for me?"

Oh my God, he's throwing me a lifeline.

"Whatever your current salary, I can top it," he continued.

The position would be salaried. I wouldn't have to worry about being on soft money. *This is too good to be true... I won't have to grovel for my very livelihood.*

Mihaelis had hired Ken Culver, MD to head the group that was to be based in Florham Park, New Jersey, and he invited me to interview for a position there. They hired me to educate and liaise with the teams conducting clinical trials to test the safety and effectiveness of the company's drugs. Together Ken and I became the "Pharmacogenetics Annex." I undertook my new challenge, blind to the cultural differences between academia and industry.

At the medical school our clinical department had had a strong research component and many PhD's. In industry, however, the usual location for someone with a PhD is within drug development research. Working with the physicians who ran the drug trials, Ken and I were far removed from those basic researchers. In that setting, having a PhD was less useful than an MD. I came to learn this the hard way.

Ken and I might have gotten along fine, and I thought that I could have gotten along with Mihaelis, but the triad set up a destructive dynamic that I have yet to fully understand. Unbeknownst to me, Ken and Mihaelis, both MDs, competed with each other from the beginning. I often felt like a pawn in the middle, never quite sure whom to trust. Most of the people who worked in the lab for Mihaelis were his former students. He had been their revered mentor. I came to believe that his retaining the lab in Maryland had a lot to do with his maintaining control over a separate empire within the company.

The need to ask "why" is primal for anyone who chooses to do scientific research. Indeed, training for a PhD consists of asking questions and then questioning the answers. In academia, one can pursue this up to the limit of one's ability to fund the required resources. Not so in the corporate environment as management (a.k.a., marketing) sets and adjusts its priorities at will. When priorities change one is expected to adapt without understanding why. I would invest months of valuable time and energy on a project, only to be told to drop it when the corporate focus changed.

As Mihaelis indicated to me, upper management had invested a great deal to incorporate pharmacogenetics. But, the "worker bees"—the people who conducted the company's routine clinical trials without much intellectual input—saw the addition of genetics mainly as annoying paperwork piled on top of their already over-burdened, day-to-day operations. When these clinical-trial leaders were resistant, Ken and I were charged with educating them about

137

the value of this new technology and helping them to develop the genetic-specific sections of their trials.

During a departmental meeting that was held in Villars, Switzerland in 2000, I was assigned to make a presentation to a group of clinical trial leaders who were resistant to incorporating pharmacogenetics into their trials. Ken had warned me, "They are going to eat us alive."

Such corporate gamesmanship constituted a challenge to Ken. To me, it constituted a paralyzing threat. My mouth was so dry that my presentation matted like cotton as I spoke. Then, during a separate session for only our pharmacogenetics group, Mihaelis challenged me to role-play how I would handle an interaction with a member of a clinical team. I self-consciously bungled a response. Ken finally "rescued" me, substituting his pharmacy fellow who proceeded to wow Mihaelis with cleverness. Outdone by a mere student, I felt humiliated. In retrospect I realize that the incident in Switzerland likely began the demise of my six-year career with Novartis.

Several years into the pharmacogenetics program, Mihaelis brought his Maryland people to New Jersey for a meeting. Ken and I sat along one side of the shiny, walnut conference table with our two assistants and our secretary; Mihaelis and his team of ten sat opposite us. A projector stood aimed at the far wall.

Managing our ever-increasing number of clinical trials had become progressively more difficult. I had taken the initiative to develop an interactive database that saved time by automatically filling in sections of the documents that were needed for each trial. I was feeling proud of what I had accomplished and was eager to show it off.

"Your database is gonna really impress them," Ken assured me.

I proceeded with my power-point presentation, anticipating the accolades that I would receive for my initiative and organization.

Mihaelis was anything but impressed. In front of the entire group he demanded, "Why did you do this without consulting me?"

"But, we discussed it last month and you agreed it was a great idea. We've already found it is saving a lot of time in generating the documents that we need for the trials."

"You didn't call me to ask how you should do it."

Misinterpreting his demeanor, I responded with a misguided attempt at finessing, "Come on, Mihaelis, I'm helping you here. I thought you'd appreciate my initiative."

"Not only are you not helping, you are in grave danger of being fired!"

No one had ever threatened me like that. I was dumbfounded, mortified. Nothing had prepared me for hand-to-hand combat with such behavior. As the gravity of his statement began to dawn, I wanted to flee the room, escape the onslaught.

Ken stepped in to deflect the now venomous attack. "Alice has single-handedly developed something which has been very helpful to us here." When Mihaelis showed no signs of relenting, Ken added, "Alice, let me talk with Mihaelis. Why don't you four go up to my office and I'll meet you there."

No one uttered a word as we trudged upstairs in disbelief. When Ken finally joined us, he reported that even Mihaelis's loyal followers had confided that they were embarrassed at his cruelty. "I can't understand what got into him," one of them told Ken. "He was definitely out of line treating Alice like that."

After the database incident, Ken engaged less enthusiastically in our activities. "We, in the PG annex, are considered second-class citizens and will never be regarded as anything more than sample collectors," he told me one day.

Ken was to leave his position soon thereafter and transfer to head another department within the company. There he controlled the pharmacogenetics being done independently of the Maryland operation. At the same time he kept abreast of Mihaelis's maneuvering. Ken's new department thrived, and Ken thrived with it.

Naively, I thought that with the triangle broken I might salvage my relationship with Mihaelis. I diligently assumed Ken's responsibilities in addition to my own. I dug in and worked all the harder in a vain attempt to please. Now a team of four in New Jersey, we needed help desperately. When the Maryland group sent us résumés of several applicants, I set up interviews for two of the candidates. We particularly liked one candidate and recommended that she be interviewed in Maryland. Once again my initiative incurred Mihaelis's wrath. "If you interview her, she'll think you're her boss," he chastised my impudence. However, several months later, when it became his choice, he hired the same candidate that we had favored.

Like Ken, I began to realize that I could not play the game according to Mihaelis's rules. By this time, though, Ken was assuring me that Mihaelis was not playing the game according to company rules. Then finally, after months and months of waiting, Ken told me, "They're relocating the Maryland group. Mihaelis was given the choice to move or leave. He's leaving."

The company subsequently restructured all of pharmacogenetics and I attempted to realign myself with this new group, even offering to relocate. But, I was told, "We really need people trained with the latest technologies." While earning my PhD, I had had exposure only to the limited repertoire of lab skills involved in gene mapping. And, by then, I was sixty-two.

Having won the respect of a physician in our Neurosciences department, I saw an opportunity to reinvent myself once again. I transferred to his department and tried to carve out a role as Neurosciences' pharmacogenetic liaison in which I assisted clinical trial leaders with the genetic component of their trial design. However, with the restructuring of pharmacogenetics, an internal departmental liaison was not considered as important as having someone who actually could run a clinical trial.

I was designated to be one of the worker bees and assigned to run the trial of a drug being re-formulated for Parkinson disease. I felt sick at heart thinking of the outlay of money and the human resources expended to reformulate a drug, not because it would be uniquely beneficial to physicians or patients, but to extend the life of its patent. I felt like I was no longer contributing to science, but to the perpetuation of Big Pharma's machine.

The newly hired MD directing the trial suggested that my lack of experience running clinical trials would jeopardize her trial. She preferred someone who had already run a trial. In academia I was respected and supported as a capable, independent researcher. In the corporate world, I simply marched in step to upper management's orders. I had once enjoyed the camaraderie of colleagues, the stimulation of lectures, the interaction with world-renowned researchers, the opportunity to teach fledgling medical students and to impact patients' lives. In Big Pharma I passed day after monotonous day with no end point in sight and no satisfaction to be had as a direct result of my efforts.

For twenty-five years I had worked in genetics at a time during which the Human Genome Project's effort to identify every human gene had made genetics a household word. I had completed my PhD at age fifty-five and made some exciting research contributions along the way. Now, I had descended to a struggle just to prove myself worthy of keeping my job. In the past, I eagerly anticipated receiving *Science* magazine, each issue brimming with something new and exciting in genetics. Now, the very sight of the magazine only triggered painful tears of longing for something lost.

At the London meeting where I had witnessed Michael J. Fox being imitated, I identified more with the patients who were being discussed than I did with the scientists doing the discussing. I had returned from the meeting traumatized by the impersonal nature of those clinical discussions, and frightened that my identity was

141

hurtling toward its own demise. My career as a scientist felt as if it were in free fall.

The work environment aside, overwhelming fatigue had made it difficult for me to keep up with the physical and intellectual demands of a full time job. Only after succumbing to the inevitable and handing my letter of resignation to Human Resources, did I charge into Enrique's office with the news. The neurologist and confidant who had confirmed the symptoms that led to my diagnosis now urged me to consider an alternative.

From behind his desk, he directed, "You're disabled, Alice. Get your letter back from HR."

"Look at me, Enrique," I protested, standing tall. "I'm not disabled, only frustrated and exhausted."

He had to repeat his message several times before I could understand, perhaps accept, what he was telling me. I did not want to be "disabled," to face all that the word implied. But, Enrique was offering me a different perspective. Why shouldn't I take advantage of the disability that our company offered its employees?

Stress may not cause Parkinson disease, but I'm convinced it can aggravate the condition. I have no doubt that the emotional toll of my humiliating experience with Big Pharma was a factor in the progression of my symptoms. After Enrique's rescue, I was placed on short-term disability. Short-term disability then became long-term disability. I was glad to be free of job related stress, and my tremor lessened appreciably. It is a bitter realization, however, that Parkinson's prevents me from being able to redeem myself in a position elsewhere, and that I will never again be an active contributor to the field that I love so much.

Chapter XIX
ON MY OWN

"You and Bob should buy a duplex so you each have your separate spaces," my friend Moni had suggested when she met my husband and witnessed our interactions. I laughed at the absurdity of her suggestion, but faced with retirement, I could no longer escape into work or school as I had done for so many years. I came to realize the kernel of wisdom in my friends' suggestion, and that it is okay for two people to care for each other and yet not be compatible living together.

It was a small incident that precipitated my leaving my marriage, not worth the re-telling. But, after forty-three years of "incidents" what finally gave me the courage to leave? I had just been given a death sentence. I had endured the demise of a wonderful career. What was the remainder of my life going to be about? At some level we are all conscious of our immortality, but we choose to distract ourselves with the business of living. Having a prognosis that spelled out that mortality made me acutely aware of just how finite is our time here on earth, and with that, came a reprioritizing of how I choose to spend that time.

I had to acknowledge the very different ways that Bob and I dealt with life. But I also knew, with great certainty, that I would eventually need someone to care for me on a daily basis. I would have expected that person to be my spouse of many years.

"How can Dad care for you if he can't care for himself?" my son asked me one day.

His simple question reverberated, and played over and over in my mind. When I became the one in need, would Bob be up to the challenge? Bob had always been there for me emotionally, yet I had

143

paid a high price in other realms. When I think back on my life's expectations, they were simple, I wanted a family, children, and a husband who would consistently nurture them and provide for us. I wanted someone who shared my values, one who would responsibly plan for a modest, but secure financial future. Certainly there were times when Bob did nurture our children, as he nurtured me, but those times were not at all predictable. I could never rely on them.

But, I could rely on me!

🕊

In August 2006, two years after being diagnosed, I moved out of our home of almost forty years and found a unit in a condominium complex that I rented for a year. I liked it! I felt exhilarated, just as I had while living in Philadelphia. I enjoyed the freedom to control my own activities. Without the constant uncertainty about Bob's mood *de-jour*, I was able to entertain friends. His lack of responsibility no longer kept me lying awake nights worrying for my future.

Bob, too, seemed happier to be living alone. Not being enmeshed constantly, we were more tolerant of each other's idiosyncrasies whenever we did share time together.

We've subsequently divorced, and I purchased a lovely condo. When friends ask, "Where are you vacationing this year?," I am surprised, as I feel I'm vacationing right here.

"Alice and Bob go on dates," my sister will tell friends who stand in awe of the fact that we have remained cordial. We have had a lifetime together, and to this day when something happens that I'm bursting to share, it is most often Bob whom I think to call.

And who will take care of me when I require assistance with daily living?

My answer is, "I really don't know." But when it happens, I know I will be able to rely on the people around me to help me figure it out—people whom I've loved and who love me.

Chapter XX
"GRAVESTONE"

In 1924 the New Jersey State Lunatic Asylum was renamed Greystone Park Psychiatric Hospital after the grey granite-like gneiss that was quarried on site and used in its construction. For me, however, the drab edifice had always conjured images of Victorian-era mistreatment of hapless souls. I pictured tortured bodies chained to beds, bruised and subsisting on bread and water. I pictured ice picks penetrating eye sockets as lobotomy patients were barbarically mutilated.

Woody Guthrie no doubt shared my impression of the place, albeit more humorously. Between 1956 and 1961, the famous balladeer was hospitalized at Greystone with Huntington disease. Sprawled on the lawn one day enjoying a visit with Bob Dylan, Woody is reputed to have dubbed his gruesome home, "Gravestone."

When it was built in the 1870s, Greystone was to be the Victorian era's remedy for appalling mental health care. With its series of connecting underground tunnels and rails, the asylum was designed as a self-contained community

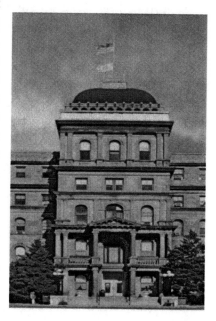

Greystone's Kirkbride facade

145

with a post office, fire and police stations, a working farm, gas and water utilities, and its own quarry. Upon opening in 1876, it accommodated 600 patients. Each ward of twenty had just two patients per "light and airy" room, its own dining room, exercise room, and parlor furnished with comfortable furniture, pianos, pictures, curtains, and fresh flowers. This idyllic description is hard for me to reconcile with what I had experienced there.

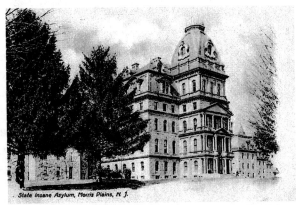

State Insane Asylum, Morris Plains, N. J.

As it turns out, Woody Guthrie was a resident at Greystone the first time I visited. Back in the spring of 1961, when I was a junior in college, Sister Anna Catherine had decided Greystone was a good place to take her Saint Elizabeth "girls" on a field trip. Several fellow biology majors aspired to become physicians, and I guess that Anna Cat saw our trip as a productive exposure to the medical profession. I had no such aspirations, for I was sure I could not stomach a medical school's first-year requisite autopsy.

"Girls, today at Greystone you are going to get to meet Dr. Morris," Sister told us before we left. "Dr. Morris has just saved a patient's life, praise God. The patient was burned over more than eighty percent of his body. No one is supposed to survive with that extensive a burn."

And, Anna Cat thinks God did the guy a favor?

Fifteen of us girls piled into three cars for the twenty-minute drive to Greystone. Anna Cat's assistant, Sister Marie Irma, accompanied us. Marie Irma was closer in age to us girls—chronologically and emotionally—than to the austere, grey-haired Sister Anna Catherine. Marie Irma dutifully spent her time providing support for us in the various laboratories. She would scurry to get agar so that we could grow bacterial plates in Microbiology, make sure that we had blades for the microtome in order to slice tissues for Histology, and at the end of the day, she'd put everything in the autoclave to be sterilized so that we could do it all again. The stiff, wimpled habit of the Sisters of Charity could not mask the impishness of her smile and manner. She had laughed as hard as we did when we came in one morning, after a careless late night in the Genetics lab, to find hundreds of fruit flies escaped from their flasks. Never mind that we had lost hours of time, and had to redo our entire experiment, she connived with us to open the windows and expunge the evidence before Anna Cat returned.

I rode to Greystone in Sr. Marie Irma's car. A driving rain commanded her concentration and stifled her usual chattiness until we arrived. "Wow, that's one big building," she exclaimed as we approached. I was tickled to be on a field trip and to spend downtime with Sr. Marie Irma. But, I was not tickled at the prospect of being at Greystone. I did not want to hear the screams of madness. The Kirkbride building towered menacingly, its weathered green dome casting an ominous shadow, even on a sunless day. Vine tendrils crept up the gloomy walls and penetrated through broken windows. Floor upon floor stood mute, unable to speak of the horrors I envisioned within their walls.

"By the late 1940's there were over 7,000 patients here," Sister Marie Irma told us. "This was one of the few places able to provide Electro-Convulsive Therapy and Insulin-Shock Therapy for the postwar trauma victims of World War Two." Her mini-history lesson did nothing to quell my revulsion.

Piling out of the cars, we scurried for the shelter of the portico. Taking the lead, Sr. Anna Catherine asked the receptionist to announce our arrival and inquired as to where we might leave coats and umbrellas. "There's a cloak room down the hall on your right, Sister."

I felt chilled by the dingy gloom and asked to hold on to my raincoat. "Girls, we don't want to drag our wet clothes into Dr. Morris's patient's room," Anna Cat directed, and I dutifully relinquished my coat.

Suddenly I felt a gust of air as an imposing figure with an extra large white coat on his six-foot frame rushed down the hallway toward us. "Sister," Dr. Morris greeted her with an outstretched hand, barely breaking stride. "How lovely to see you and your girls." Here was a physician who would have no trouble getting unruly patients to cooperate. "I understand that some of these young ladies are going to be doctors." He knew Sister's soft spot. "Have we any psychiatrists in the group?"

"Yes," Sister beamed. "Mary Lynn here, and Theresa have expressed interest. Theresa's father is a well known thoracic surgeon at Columbia in New York." For a humble nun, Anna Cat was mighty adept at aligning with status. "I'm sure whatever you show the girls will be useful in their scientific careers."

But, I only want to do research. I don't want to see a patient with more than half his skin missing. What if his face is gone?

"Follow Dr. Morris, girls." Lemming-like, I followed the crowd. The unpleasant scent of stale urine permeated the air. Marching down the dulled hospital-green halls amidst stalactites of ceiling paint, I paused to glimpse through a small high window into one of the closed doors lining the hallway. The room was deserted, but jail-like bars on the outside would have assured any patient's stay. I shuddered, looked away, and scurried after the crowd.

"My patient is in the room ahead to our left," Dr. Morris boomed. "He is a fifty-two year old male who disobeyed the rules a month ago by smoking in bed. His mattress caught on fire, and by the time I saw him, I didn't think we were going to be able to save him. I did skin grafting, but some areas are just bandaged and will have to await the growth of new skin. We have to change his dressings and treat the wounds daily to prevent infection."

He stopped by a door and turned the knob. "Michael, can you hear me?" he asked, throwing open the door so that we could all flood in. "I've brought some beautiful young ladies to see you."

Michael uttered a low moan. Shrouded from head to toe, he could have been Boris Karloff's mummy, for all of him that was identifiable.

Michael must be just thrilled to be surrounded by a bevy of women. At least his face is covered so he can't see us gawking at him.

"Michael, I'm going to sit you up now," Dr. Morris warned. As the mummy was raised to a sitting position its moan became more audible. "Michael, I need to change this bandage on your back, and I want to show these ladies how well you're doing." As he peeled back the red-tinged gauze, tiny pieces of stuck flesh pulled with it. I felt the rawness of the graft, and Michael cried out in agony.

Suddenly, I felt my consciousness peel away, and I struggled to reach the door before passing out. Sr. Marie Irma grabbed my arm and must have summoned a nurse who appeared with smelling salts. My field trip was over. Marie Irma came with me to retrieve our coats and we waited for the others in the car.

"I'm so embarrassed," I cried. "Anna Cat will think I'm a bloody chicken!"

"A very compassionate bloody chicken," she said, her hand resting gently on mine.

Twenty-five years after my initial visit to Greystone my work with Huntington's patients took me there once again. It was not without trepidation. The memory of my first visit to that dismal place can still send a chill up my spine. Rita, the mother of one of my patients in Greystone, had phoned me one day to express distress about her daughter's care. "Rosemary is being treated like an animal at Greystone. She spends her days on the floor in a hallway because they lock her room behind her, and when she smokes she gets burns all over her body. They don't know anything about caring for

Huntington disease. Can't you visit the staff and show them how they need to treat these patients?"

Rita had already lost a son to HD and, because a private alternative was prohibitively expensive, she was now forced to witness her daughter's inhumane treatment in a facility equipped to managing psychotic masses simply by doling out huge quantities of anti-psychotic drugs. How ironic to find that the Greystone staff was clueless about the illness suffered by their most famous patient, Woody Guthrie.

"I am so sorry to hear about what's happening to Rosemary. It has to be sheer torture for you to see. I will make an appointment to talk with the staff about her care as soon as I can."

During the end stages of Huntington's, patient management becomes increasingly difficult, and placement in an institution often becomes necessary. Behavioral manifestations of the disorder—psychosis, uncontrolled anger, and disinhibition—frequently land these patients in psychiatric hospitals. As coordinator of the HD Family Service Center, I taught staff at various long-term facilities about the needs of HD patients and advocated for care that accommodated the patient's physical deterioration.

Another rainy day, approaching the campus, the Kirkbride building loomed as huge and menacing to me as it had when I was a student. Once again the angst that I felt outside the building paled by comparison to the horror I found inside. But, I had work to do. I had to suppress any queasiness and focus on my mission. I had brought a slide presentation on HD care that I delivered whenever a facility requested help in managing patients in their charge. I had to find a way to improve things for my young patient. Rosemary was only twenty-five and already well into the typical fifteen to twenty year course of the disease.

"Hi, I'm Ms. Lazzarini and I'm here to do the in-service on HD," I said, reaching to shake the hand of the aide who had unlocked the door to let me in. (In 1988 I had not yet earned the title, Dr.)

"Glad you came. We sure need some teachin' 'bout this disease."

I found myself immediately in a "common room." It was actually a cavernous hallway, with some thirty or so patients, men and women, in various stages of disarray. Low-wattage, bare bulbs hugged the ceiling, many burned out. The hospital-green walls were unchanged, perhaps unpainted, since my visit twenty-five years before. Again, there was the vague, musty odor. I wanted to turn and run. Some patients looked at me, curious. Most were oblivious. Somehow, each had adapted to the inevitability of living in his or her dark, dingy dungeon of a home—to life at Gravestone. I saw only one attendant, and hoped that none of these patients was dangerous.

"Before I start my talk," I asked, "could you show me where to find Rosemary?"

"She's right there," the aide said, pointing down the hall to a heap lying on the bare tile floor.

"My God," I uttered, unable to fathom their treating anyone with less respect than I might afford an animal. She was dressed in a scanty, summer-weight dress, and was curled into a fetal position, her still body pressed against the wall. She must have been asleep, for only then—and in the very last stages of the disease—do HD patients get relief from their constant movements.

"Rosemary," I said, gently touching her shoulder.

She opened her eyes and looked up. She had known me from many visits to our clinic, but she showed no sign of recognition. She was shivering and cold to the touch, her dress disheveled, her hair matted. As her arms and legs began to writhe, I saw that she had at least twenty reddish purple scars and singed hairs from burning cigarette ashes having fallen on her bare skin. I let her return to the blessed reprieve of sleep.

Incredulous, I asked, "Why isn't Rosemary in her bed?"

"Safety says we have to lock bedroom doors during the day, so all the patients be out here where we can seeum."

"But she has end-stage Huntington's. She really needs to be able to rest!"

"Can't break rules in this place ya' know."

"She's shivering. Why isn't she at least dressed warmly or given a blanket?"

"Don't got extras. If you're ready, you can follow me."

She led me down the hall and used her key to let us through another locked door. I felt a modicum of protection with the patients locked behind us, but I longed to bring Rosemary to safety with me. We entered an unadorned room furnished with standard-issue tables and straight-back chairs. A small microwave, coffee machine, and mini-refrigerator told me that I was in the staff lunchroom.

As I set up my laptop, eight or nine staff members ambled in. They listened attentively and asked questions about the disease that had landed Rosemary in their midst. Well meaning as they were, they were limited in what they could do within a system whose supplies and resources were stretched so thinly. I did convince them that Rosemary was well beyond the point of being a danger to herself or others in the psychiatric sense, and that she needed access to her bedroom to rest during the day.

Cigarettes are a formidable problem with HD patients as the uncontrolled movements make connecting the cigarette with the lighter a challenge. Flicking ashes then becomes random. Like food, however, smoking becomes a last bastion when all of life's other pleasures have been stripped away. Deciding when it is time for a smoke also becomes a last bastion of control, the loss of which can result in an angry, very insistent HD patient. Rosemary's cigarettes were to be kept locked at the nurse's station and smoking was to be supervised -WHEN and IF there was a staff member available.

I have to find another facility that will take Rosemary.

It was her mother who found one of those rare nursing homes that took a Medicaid patient without a prior payment. I gave a similar presentation there to a staff eager to deliver proper care. Shortly thereafter, Rosemary died in her bed. She had, at least, spent her last days surrounded by people who were committed to maintaining her dignity.

Chapter XXI
THE MONSTER IS GONE

There had long been talk of demolishing Greystone's aging physical plant after the county took it over from the state. Then one day driving back to my home after visiting Bob, I took a shortcut through the grounds of Greystone Park Psychiatric Hospital. The road curved a bit differently around new construction, and suddenly a sun-drenched, unobstructed skyline struck me. The imposing Kirkbride building that had towered ominously against the heavens was nowhere in sight.

"Oh, my God, the monster is gone," I exclaimed out loud to myself.

"My God, the monster really is gone!" I repeated, even louder, feeling relief at the obliteration of some horror. The intensity of my response surprised me. What, exactly, did that monster represent to invoke such a dramatic reaction?

There were times when I would have equated the monster with my marraige, times when I felt oppressed, chained to a bed of my own making, confined to a prison from which I couldn't leave. The building that, years earlier, had frightened me to the point of immobility was gone at the exact point in time that I had managed to break free from that bondage.

But, the monster went farther back than that. I could finally declare to my deceased mother, "You never were able to demand your right to be treated with consideration, and you taught me subservience. But, I have learned that I have the right to insist that people treat me with respect." And, I can at long last proclaim to my late father, "Your over-protecting me didn't make me safer; it made me more vulnerable and less able to feel self sufficient. But, I no longer need protection; I am strong and I can protect myself."

My exaltation had everything to do with my own bravery. I had once stood by the mummy's bed, a witness to his pain yet, in that moment, feeling transfixed, powerless to relieve it. So, too, had I once felt powerless to make changes in my own life, my moment of immobility enduring for years. The monster that I had shed was the emotional dependency that was my lifelong companion. I had cast off painful shyness and anxiety and claimed the power to be true to myself and to face my own future.

Not long thereafter, I once again cut through Greystone Park. The familiar Victorian facade loomed up on the distant hill to my left.

"Damn, the monster is still there," I blurted, crestfallen.

Maneuvering through the new construction, I had been looking in the wrong direction, at the wrong skyline. The Greystone monster was definitely still there. Somehow, though, it did not look quite as imposing that day in the sunlight.

So too, the Parkinson disease monster remains. I face a predictable decline in my ability to stand tall and in my ability to take care of myself. One day I may be unable to advocate for myself as I once had advocated for Rosemary. I, too, may find myself in an institution at the mercy of strangers, as was Michael. But, having been diagnosed with a disease that foreshadows such utter dependency, I know deep within me how precious is the gift of time. Devoid of the illusion that I have forever to figure it all out, I find myself acutely aware of wanting to get every day right. I can choose whether to spend my time compromising who I am, or I can fully partake of the person who I was born to be.

When I was first diagnosed, I had refused participation in a drug trial. I had not been ready then to allow Parkinson's into my life. But now, Parkinson's not only limits my productivity to a few hours per day, it has distorted my sense of smell so that the roses in my garden lack fragrance, or sometimes I will smell pungent odors that are not there. I will sit on my trembling hand so as not to call attention to my condition, or to prevent any untoward movement from knocking my dentist's hand. Friends will ask me to repeat myself when my lowering voice can't be heard, and I have trouble rolling over in bed. My computer mouse clicks without intent and, when I write out something longhand, I am shocked at how deteriorated my script has become. I occasionally lose my balance and am unnerved when I have to seize something in order to support myself. These things have so far been manageable with a smattering of patience and a dollop of humor.

Nevertheless, I can envision a day when I might choose to bet everything I have on the chance that some new treatment might forestall my increasingly debilitating symptoms and allow me to continue enjoying my life.

I don't want to miss feeling an overwhelming sense of pride "working the room," when my son has his first solo show at the Museum of Modern Art.

I don't want to miss feeling excited as I stand and cheer for my granddaughter playing drums in her first rock concert, and throwing a lavish party when she becomes engaged to the love of her life.

I don't want to miss the delight of calling all the newspapers with an announcement about my nephew opening his own business, and being able to dance at his wedding.

I don't want to miss the pleasure of distributing journal reprints when my grandson's first contribution to science is published.

I don't want Parkinson disease to rob me of movement so that I am no longer able to hug my daughter and tell her how very much I love her.

I don't want Parkinson's to cause the muscles in my face to mask, so that I can no longer smile.

I want to always be able to laugh.

When these things are threatened, will I say "yes" to someone doing something so radical as taking my skin cells, transforming them into PARKINSON'S-killing machines and shooting them back into my brain?

You bet I will.

And, when that chess master declares "checkmate," and Parkinson disease finally is conquered, I will have the satisfaction of knowing that I had been a key player in the glorious game of science that was the genetics of Parkinson disease.

Chapter XXII
Coping With Parkinson Disease

It would feel presumptive for me to prescribe a way for someone else to cope with Parkinson disease. Each of us has our own unique set of coping skills that we bring to bear when diagnosed with a condition that is "neurodegenerative."

In general I lean toward depression. I've been on a maintenance dose of antidepressants since losing my mother twenty years ago, and few things during that time have pushed me to despair. Yet, today I feel the anguish of loss witnessing the decline of our beloved "Boss." The story of the discovery of PARK1 and *alpha-synuclein* would not have unfolded as it did without Roger Duvoisin. This man, who had the courage to reverse his own conviction, changed the paradigm of existing PD dogma and precipitated a research revolution. Now, nearing ninety years of age, his gait is shuffled, his posture stooped, his days spent mostly alone. He reads avidly yet his conversation is predominantly reminiscent, and World War II stories seem fresher in his memory than recollections of his own considerable contributions to science. Still self-aware that a medical evaluation showed, "I am no longer safe to be driving," and "my kids have taken over my finances," he seems sad but resolute. I admire his courage; I ache at the indignity he endures.

So, how graciously will I accept my own projected decline? Interestingly, my inspiration comes not from the time I spent researching Parkinson's but from my eleven years of intimate interaction with Huntington disease families. Parkinson's and Huntington's are both movement disorders and have been referred to as mirror images. While Parkinson's patients typically have trouble moving, Huntington's patients have trouble stopping their excess dance-like movements or dyskinesias. And these are the same dyskinesias that are seen in Parkinson's patients as a side effect of medications that are needed in order just to be able to move at all.

Today researchers recognize an increasing commonality among neurodegenerative disorders in that each is characterized by protein clumps that wreak havoc in the brain. But, there are also commonalities in the burden that a slow, agonizing deterioration puts on an individual and his or her entire family, as affirmed in our coining the "Huntington Disease Family Service Center." As the program's coordinator, I was the first point of contact for families in distress. I soon realized that what they needed was someone to listen, someone to care that a loved one was just jailed because a cop mistook his uncontrolled flailing for drunkenness, or that there was no place to keep Mom safe from harm while son or daughter had to work. I helped people get medical alert bracelets or to find suitable care facilities, but I also ran a summer camp program for the patients themselves.

A colleague of mine convinced the folks at the Vacation Camp for the Blind in Suffern, New York to share their facilities for the weeklong pilot program that we proposed for five HD campers. I felt grateful not to have to explain to the many sightless campers with whom we shared the facilities why our patients were in constant motion. But the true genius of the plan revealed itself one day with a camper named Donna. She had arrived from upstate New York with her young husband and three little children. Her needs were such that her husband essentially had four children. Devoted to his wife, scared for her future and scared for his kids, of all the caretakers he was most in need of the week's respite. Yet he was the last to leave, needing our reassurance that Donna would do well in our care. Indeed she sensed that, immediately bid them all farewell, and bounded into her new adventure. She was really in love with Huey Lewis, she confided to me.

I escorted Donna to cabin number three, where we would bunk together and she would keep up a weeklong running dialogue. No subject was off limits. She described to me the horror of having lived through her father's decline, and knew full well the trajectory that she faced. One day we strolled together through camp, Donna writhing so uncontrollably that I marveled that she could remain upright. Our conversation was interrupted when we came upon a blind camper. Pausing to process the man's disability, she drew me close and whispered as if in confidence, "Thank God I can see." There are infinite poignant moments that I treasure from our exhausting, weeklong immersion in the chaos, flailing, and disinhibition that is Huntington disease, but Donna's perspective on her disability is my perpetual inspiration.

I lived with families shattered by the complexities of Huntington's: the guilt of having passed the disease to one's children, the frustration of managing a loved one who has slipped into psychosis, the complete draining of financial and emotional resources, yet I also witnessed heroics.

Stu Faden and Sam Baily shared a bond that few of us experience. Each watched a parent die in an asylum for the insane, shriveled and incoherent. Stu and Sam lived everyday with the knowledge that they had a 50% risk of developing the disorder that had destroyed their parents before there was widespread understanding of their unique needs. Both men were married to loving women who shared that fear with them. Both of their wives had learned that if a cure wasn't developed in time, the disease could also destroy their children, born before either one even knew what HD was. I had seen such marriages left strewn like broken boards after a karate tournament. But Stu and Sam and their wives gathered up the pieces and turned their fear into a cause. They became activists for the Huntington's Disease Society of America (HDSA), volunteering their time in all manner of fund raising endeavors. Together they became the face of the families, as well as the support behind our HD Family Service Center.

One day Stu said to me, "Alice, if they can have a summer camp for HD patients in Canada, we should do it here in New Jersey. After all, everyone looks to you for ideas on providing services for HD." He wanted to provide respite for HD caretakers, and he wanted to enable HD patients to forestall HD's downward trajectory. For one week at least, they could have an experience that would set them free.

"Great idea," I told him. From that moment on, New Jersey's HD camp was a *fait accompli.*

I'd like to tell you that for their altruism, each was spared the burden of HD, but alas, no. The founder of what became the Samuel L. Baily Huntington Disease Family Service Center did not inherit the disease-causing gene and he continues to enjoy life with his wife, three children and seven grandchildren in the knowledge that they are spared the agony of HD. His being spared is not without burden, however, as he watches his dear friend Stu slowly ravaged by the disease. A staunch advocate of a healthy diet, Stu's disease initially progressed so slowly that physicians cited him as an example of a "model patient." Now he is wheel chair bound, virtually incoherent, and totally dependent. Stu's wife, a former career executive, now lives the life of a full-time caregiver, devoted to maintaining dignity for the man she and so many of us love, buoyed only by the reassurance that predictive testing showed her child to be free of the disease-causing gene.

When I recently had surgery to repair the rotator cuff in my left shoulder, I worried about all the usual things surrounding a surgical procedure. But, when the procedure was over I was surprised to realize the extent to which I had to rely on friends and family to shower me, to dress me, to prepare food, even feed me as I am left-handed and inept at using my right hand. I came closer to despair than I have experienced since being diagnosed with PD, and realized the degree to which I am frightened of being dependent. I have fought so hard to achieve my independence, planted my flag in the sand and declared, in the words of Helen Reddy, "I am woman, hear me roar..." Now, what frightens me most about the advancing course of Parkinson's is reaching the point whereby I must depend, like Roger, like Donna, and like Stu, on the generosity of others.

Then I heard of reporter Miles O'Brien's freak accident that resulted in the loss of his left arm. Scarcely a month later, he was reporting on CNN as an aviation expert regarding the loss of Malaysia's flight 370. As I sat in pain that promised to be short-lived, I heard him describe his never-ending phantom limb pain. I looked deep into his eyes as if to penetrate the TV and partake of his fortitude. He's already joked on his blog about "playing the hand that one is dealt," and I'm reminded of another source of inspiration from my Huntington days. Nancy Wexler was a prime force behind the field trip to Venezuela to study a family that, in 1983, would result in locating the causative HD gene. Herself at 50% risk for inheriting the disease, she would affirm her own coping strategy saying, "it is not the hand you're dealt, but how you play that hand that matters." I draw now on the examples of Nancy and all those who have impacted my life in a profound way, from Roger's gentility in facing the loss of basic activities, to Donna's perspective on her condition relative to others, to Stu's wife's fortitude in preserving her husband's dignity.

So, what to do with my fear of dependence? It is a battle I wage every day, but one that I am determined to win. I have dutifully adhered to my physical therapy regimen in an effort to regain complete function of my dominant arm. I aim to get back to regularly doing early morning walks and reinstating my gym membership because I know it helps my mood, but also because exercise has been proven to have benefit in forestalling the decline of Parkinson's. I challenge my mind playing bridge and scrabble, serve on the board of my townhouse association, and keep engaged with my friends.

Another lesson driven home by my HD families is an appreciation of the amount of energy that is expended to protect a secret. The woman who was hit with the news that she was at 50% risk for Huntington's on the eve of her wedding in a misguided attempt at protecting her from the hereditary nature of her father's disease, and then she in turn hid it from her spouse until after they had children and she became symptomatic, was a sure recipe for disaster.

But, I also saw families that chose to discuss HD openly, without shame—as needed, similar to the "sex talk"—and this approach produced far healthier, well-adjusted children. Granted, fear of losing one's job or otherwise being discriminated against certainly justifies caution in some arenas. I have had the good fortune to be able to be open and honest about my PD diagnosis since I retired on disability. If one is able to be candid about the condition from the onset, explaining to those who care for you why you have a tremor, stumble a bit, or stare with a blank expression, you relieve a certain awkwardness on their part and people tend to respond with compassion, not pity. You also offer them the opportunity to more easily accommodate your changes over time.

Because Parkinson's progresses slowly, one is faced with constantly confronting change—a new awareness with the loss of each piece of your former self. Pain and sorrow inevitably occur as the ability to do what once was easy, decreases. Pity parties are allowed. Give in and feel it. Then try to accept the new reality, determine what you can still do and find some enjoyment in each new day.

Linda, a former model and the first HD patient whom I saw, was, at twenty-nine, already too disabled to keep up with her secretarial job. I remember counseling her to separate the two main reasons that we go to work each day: to earn a living and to derive satisfaction in feeling useful. She had the first covered with disability payments, so we worked on the myriad of ways she might fulfill the second. Hearing my own counsel, I find satisfaction now in my garden and the persistence of the perennials that appear year after year. I find satisfaction, too, in sharing my experiences with the hope of helping others with Parkinson's.

Of all the times to be living with Parkinson's, now is the most hopeful of times. Prior to our 1997 discovery of the role of *alpha-*

synuclein in Parkinson's, doctor's simplistically attempted to appease the diseased brain by replacing its missing dopamine. Now, akin to the Human Genome Project that was aimed at mapping each of our genes, the BRAIN Initiative (Brain Research through Advancing Innovative Neurotechnologies) aims at mapping the activity of each of our brain cells. Launched in 2013 with approximately $100 million, and with additional support from the private sector, scientists at NIH will study how the brain operates in both healthy and diseased states, map out the brain's neural networks and unravel how they interrelate in an attempt to help researchers find new ways to treat, cure, and even prevent disorders like Parkinson's. And, because Parkinson's progresses slowly, you have every right to maintain the hope—as I do—that researchers will make further exponential progress in our lifetime.

Keep the faith.

Lastly, I remember my mom surviving the loss of her spouse of close to fifty years and then her eyesight to Macular Degeneration. Yet, she never complained.

"Your mom was one of the bravest people I know," Bob has told me frequently.

And where did that courage to soldier on come from? It has to come from deep within. When you doubt or despair, try calling to mind someone to emulate, someone whose courage you can absorb into your own core. Whether you meditate or pray, do avail yourself of the power of someone's healing.

As my mom did, I would like to leave my family, not with memories of my having been bitter, but with respect for my courage. Her example of being brave in the face of loss was a generous gift that I would share with each of you, but alas I can leave you only with her favorite prayer:

Lord, make me an instrument
of your peace,
where there is hatred, let me sow love,
where there is injury, pardon,
where there is doubt, faith,
where there is despair, hope,
where there is darkness, light,
and where there is sadness, joy.
O Divine Master,
grant that I may not so much seek
to be consoled as to console,
to be understood as to understand,
to be loved as to love.
For it is in giving that we receive,
it is in pardoning that we are pardoned,
and it is in dying that we are
born to eternal life.

Prayer of Saint Francis

And also with mine...

God grant me the serenity

to accept the things I cannot change;

the courage to change the things I can;

and the wisdom to know the difference.

POSTSCRIPT
GONE TO THE BIRDS...

I recently had the opportunity to fulfill a wish to visit the laboratory of Dr Erich Jarvis, Duke University Medical Center's award-winning neurobiologist, and to see his zebra finches in person. My instinct was still to flinch with the fluttering of wings, but it was now tempered with a feeling of gratitude to my feathered friends for continuing to inform research that contributes to our understanding of Parkinson disease.

Our close relative, the chimpanzee, has only limited ability to learn new vocalizations, but oscine songbirds that learn vocal expression, like the zebra finch and parrot, are model organisms to study parallels with human speech. Because dopamine, the neurotransmitter that is depleted in Parkinson's, is the key player in modulating the bird's song, understanding these processes at the molecular level in the songbird can greatly inform our understanding of the neuropathology involved in PD.

A male zebra finch memorizes his father's unique song and he will sing the same song for life. The 2010 sequencing of the zebra finch genome enabled comparison with the genome of the only other bird to be sequenced, the non-song-learning chicken, and this has allowed identification of genes that are unique to song learning.[1] Area X, a brain region dedicated to vocal-motor function that is present only in song-learning birds, is comparable to areas in the human basal ganglia that are responsible for dopamine release, and that are damaged in Parkinson disease. A recent review of the comparative anatomy, circuitry, and function of these structures reveals the great extent to which the songbird has informed our search for understanding of pathways that go awry in PD.[2]

Gene expression in the area of the finch's brain responsible for song has been shown to overlap with specific genes involved in processes such as synaptic function and plasticity, which are disrupted in PD.[3] One of those genes, FOXP2, has a well-established role in vocalization integral to normal human speech, and its close relative, FOXP1, is reduced in mice lacking an *alpha-synuclein* gene.[4]

"I'd like to see a mutated *alpha-synuclein* gene inserted into a songbird," I quipped to Dr. Jarvis, trying to envision what the results might be. I thought I had posed an impossible problem, as I couldn't imagine the process of inserting a foreign gene into an embryo that had a protective eggshell.

"Oh, but we are trying to making transgenic zebra finches," he told me, reflecting on the work of his colleague Fernando Nottebohm at Rockefeller University who has created a songbird that lights up with green fluorescent protein.[5]

It has been more than 15 years since our discovery that a mutation in *alpha-synuclein* causes Parkinson disease, and the mechanism by which this happens is being painstakingly deciphered. But, it *is* being deciphered, and the tiny zebra finch, with its gray striped breast and bright red beak, sings in his cage oblivious to the important role he continues to play.

Epilogue
ALPHA-SYNUCLEIN AND ME

At a departmental lecture late in the summer of 1996, Dr. Bill Nicklas and I debated our respective positions: nature vs. nurture as the cause of Parkinson disease. As we stood eye to eye, Bill smiled his gentle smile and displayed the easy confidence that comes from having contributed so much to a body of work that one knows one's place in the history of science is established, even before the book is written. I stood in awe of his stature, but that day the upstart in me felt suddenly emboldened. I had just received word from NIH that we were close to the breakthrough that was to become PARK1, and I drew an uncharacteristic line in the sand.

"You are barking up an awfully tall tree," I told Bill, firm in my support of the nature argument. "Finding a causative gene is the quickest way to understand the basic cause of Parkinson's." I would allow that environmental factors might influence the expression of a gene, but we had to find the gene—or genes—first.

"But you are not taking into account that studies consistently have shown pesticide exposure as a risk factor for Parkinson's. This points to the effect of an environmental toxin," he responded— erudite professor to impatient student. Continuing his nurture argument, he reminded me, "Our studies have clearly demonstrated that MPTP[1] kills dopamine neurons by inhibiting Complex I of the mitochondrial respiratory chain."

"We'll see…" I challenged dismissively as we took our seats in the front row.

Envisioning myself sprinting hare-like to the finish line, I was too heady with the imminence of our results from NIH to give credence to Bill's tortoise-like, methodical, long-distance pace.

169

The Department of Neurology at the Robert Wood Johnson Medical School has two arms, a clinical arm and a research arm. The clinical arm, where patients are seen, is in New Brunswick, while the research laboratories are across the Raritan River on the Piscataway campus. When department members gathered for weekly meetings or joint lectures, there was always a friendly competition between us. In the global world of Parkinson disease research, some scientists believed that it has a genetic origin (nature), while others argued that it is caused by environmental factors (nurture). Proponents on each side were willing to go to the mat in support of their theory.

Advocates of the environmental theory postulated that mitochondrial dysfunction and oxidative stress are central to the pathogenesis. Mitochondria, the tiny organelles within every cell that function in energy metabolism, are particularly plentiful in tissues like the brain that require high energy. Oxidative stress is a concept that has been brought into the popular lexicon by proponents of all those antioxidant supplements, and it refers to the toxic byproducts that are generated as cells utilize oxygen.

In the early 1980s, young drug addicts in California inadvertently provided a definitive connection between mitochondrial damage and Parkinson's symptoms. A byproduct, formed during the preparation of their designer drugs, caused a syndrome that resembled Parkinson disease and was temporarily relieved by the same medications as were used to treat Parkinson disease. As it turned out, the byproduct was the chemical, MPTP, a brain poison that inhibits mitochondria, and the pattern of cell death that it causes closely resembles the pathology of Parkinson's.

Mitochondrial damage and a mouse-model of MPTP-toxicity became the focus of the research arm of our department whose laboratories were headed by world-respected leaders in the neurosciences. Bill Nicklas and his colleague, Dick Heikkila, were among the strongest advocates of the environmental theory. Together they published a landmark paper demonstrating the way in which MPTP causes certain brain cells to die.[2] They devoted their entire research careers to working out the minute details of this

170

neurotoxicity. By 1990, when I arrived, Bill and Dick's neurosciences research group was producing paper after paper demonstrating a role for toxins in the pathogenesis of Parkinson's.

However, in the clinical arm of the department, many of us had begun to bet our chips on the nature argument. After all, we had our proof that genetics would win out over environment in the Parkinson's chess game.

Roger's identical twin pairs had him rethinking the possibility of an underlying genetic cause. The 1994 study, in which I examined disease recurrence within the families of Roger's patients, further supported a genetic component to Parkinson's. And, of course, we had identified the Contursi family. Observing that the disease passed down through multiple generations, and that approximately half of the offspring of an affected individual developed the disease, this family clearly demonstrated a single-gene inheritance pattern. After the paper describing this pedigree was published,[3] colleagues from throughout the neurology community had begun telling us of additional multi-case families.

As departmental chairman, Roger loyally supported the work done on both sides of the river, refusing to close one door upon the other. Now, research that has been done as a result of Roger's leadership in discovering the *alpha-synuclein* mutation, PARK1, has facilitated the convergence of the genetic and environmental theories, each one informing the other.

Our genetic finding validated what the environmentalists had been seeing all along. By 2001, mutations in *alpha-synuclein* had been demonstrated to interfere with the pathway that is responsible for removing damaged proteins from neurons. When mitochondrial dysfunction results in oxidative stress, proteins accumulate and interfere with the very same pathway. Nature and nurture were beginning to tell us an overlapping story.

Researchers have discovered important links between individuals with hereditary Parkinson's and those with what appears to be a sporadic form of the disease. Subsequent to our discovery of

PARK1, many other Parkinson's-causing genes have been identified, and at least 12 other genes have been implicated as in some way associated with the disease.[4] Understanding the roles that all of these genes play is beginning to clarify, not only the pathway responsible for removing damaged proteins, but multiple pathways that are at play in the disease pathogenesis (see Appendices).

In a press release dated January 4, 2008, the Michael J. Fox Foundation for Parkinson's Research announced their Linked Efforts to Accelerate Parkinson's Solutions initiative to address how *alpha-synuclein*, and another Parkinson's-implicated protein, LRRK2, trigger the death of dopamine neurons. The announcement included the following statement:

"*Alpha-synuclein* was the first gene associated with Parkinson's, and pathological clumping of the protein product of the *alpha-synuclein* gene within cells of the brain represents a nearly universal thread linking multiple forms of Parkinson's."

On January 15, 2008 another Fox Foundation press release announced $2 million in funding, under their Critical Challenges in Parkinson disease Research, for the development of a gene silencing therapeutic with which to treat Parkinson disease by reducing expression of the protein *alpha-synuclein*. That announcement included the following statement:

"More and more scientific evidence supports the hypothesis that lowering *alpha-synuclein* levels in the brain could achieve the so-called 'Holy Grail' of Parkinson's research, a neuroprotective therapy."

Does that mean that the answers are right around the corner and that we will have a cure tomorrow? Not really. Science frequently allows us to answer one question at the same time that it raises ten more. In comparison to the days in genetics when we thought linearly: one gene → one pathway → one cure, the science has become extremely complicated. Given the urgency of my personal fight against Parkinson's, the research can feel painfully slow.

I long to get back into the game and to take part in flushing out more answers, but I cannot. The excessive fatigue of Parkinson's has robbed me of my ability to work full time. Now, I must be content to speak out and to help to raise money that will ensure that the many inspired researchers whom I have known throughout my career will have the funding that it takes to move the science forward. I must have faith that they will successfully advance their chess pieces across that playing board.

But, I wonder, will they be able to sort out all the genes and their pathways quickly enough, and will the opponent's king be out-maneuvered in time to help me?

For the six years that I worked in the pharmaceutical industry, I experienced first-hand the laborious process of drug development that follows an initial discovery. The realist in me worries that an improved treatment option won't be available in time for me.

Then again, recent studies in cell-culture have begun to decipher the specific mechanism whereby *alpha-synuclein* aggregates wreak their havoc. By causing the waste-disposing lysosomes to rupture, reactive oxygen species are released, inducing mitochondrial dysfunction and inflammation.[5] It is by deciphering these pathways that treatment breakthroughs will be forthcoming.

For me, *alpha-synuclein* has come full-circle, connecting mitochondrial toxicity with genetic defects. Just maybe the nature:nurture dance that our department's beloved "Boss" choreographed will lead to a way of preventing the devastation that this disease waits to impose on me and on millions of other PD patients throughout the world.

I live in hope.

BACKWORD

by Moni Hopwood, PhD

Years ago when Alice and I had first received our diagnoses of Parkinson's disease and she first started talking about writing this book we joked about my writing a "backword." Everyone else had forewords; so Alice needed a backword. Here it is.

The parallels in our stories have never ceased to amaze me; earlier scientific research, late doctorates, forced out of academia by lack of funding, difficult careers in industry and finally, diagnoses of Parkinson's. Yet there are remarkable differences as well. While we both have Parkinson's, we still have very different diseases. I first developed signs and symptoms of PD at the age of 34, putting me into the young-onset group like Michael J Fox, but was misdiagnosed with multiple sclerosis since young-onset PD was not widely recognized at the time. When I was finally correctly diagnosed I had had the disease for almost twenty years. Alice's case is the more typical later onset PD and thus newer and less advanced than mine. There also are differences in symptom patterns and medication response. Young-onset PD tends to progress at a slower rate but responds to dopamine replacement with earlier and more severe dyskinesias (involuntary abnormal movements that get you noticed by talk show radio hosts). There are still more differences, but the end result is the same—slow debilitation related to dopamine deficiency. Still one needs to remember—each case of Parkinson's is unique because it is happening to a unique individual.

And then those parallels! Like Alice I got my PhD later in life (in my 40's) after putting in many years of medical research and yet was forced by funding difficulties into taking a job in industry. Not that there is anything wrong with industry; we just aren't suited to it, being academicians at heart. Oh, how both of us missed (and still miss) academics! My experience in industry was somewhat more positive than Alice's but we both had difficult departures. Glass ceilings are called that for good reason; one doesn't really see one until one smashes face first into it.

Alice's experiences are a clear example of a woman's difficulties in the workplace, especially given her eminent professional status prior to the move into industry. If these challenges were not enough, she faces and triumphs over personal hurdles as well. "Both Sides Now" is a story of a woman's trials in the modern work-world and home and her tribulations in overcoming them. Her introspection over these experiences should advise many young women, both in academia and in industry.

I am proud to have been part of "Both Sides Now" and prouder yet to be Alice's friend. Her story is one to be remembered.

APPENDIX I

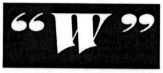

FAMILY NEWSLETTER
VOLUME 3 ❦ NUMBER 1
SPRING, 1995

ALICE LAZZARINI, M.S.
DIRECTOR CLINICAL GENETICS
DIVISION OF NEUROGENETICS
DEPARTMENT OF NEUROLOGY
UMDNJ-Robert Wood Johnson Medical School
New Brunswick, NJ 08903...(908)-235-7340

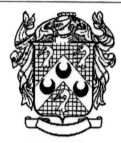

Our work...and your help has paid off. We have found the 'W' family gene! AND we have made contact with a whole new branch of the family connected by brothers who lived in the 17th Century. Not too many people can identify a 5th cousin twice removed!

We like to think of the discovery of the gene as a wedding gift for Jerry Jenkins and his lovely bride, Deana. Jerry had originally brought the family to our attention and made this research possible. He and Deana came to the dedication of our laboratory in May of 1993, along with Betsy Lovett whose husband's generous gift established the William Dow Lovett Laboratory of Neurogenetics. We wish **each** of you could have been there to share in the official ribbon cutting ceremony.

I would like to speak with **each** of you personally, and tell you what this discovery means, how it may affect you, and what we will do next. I hope this newsletter begins that process and that you will feel free to call or write to me with any questions.

If you get the newsletter, *Generations*, from the National Ataxia Foundation, you have been reading about spinocerebellar ataxia type 1 (SCA1). Persons with SCA1 have been found to have too many copies of a genetic 'word,' CAG, located within a gene on chromosome #6. We were able to rule out chromosome # 6 in the Whipple family, but there were several other locations where genes for the dominant ataxias have been found. These are being named SCA1, SCA2, SCA3.... and so on. The gene in your family is the same as that for Machado Joseph Disease (MJD), an ataxia whose name derived from the families in which it was first described.

As in SCA1, persons with MJD have too many copies of CAG, but on chromosome #14, not chromosome #6. We still do not understand how the extra copies of CAG cause the disease, or why it affects certain areas of the brain. Does finding the gene guarantee we will have a cure? The answer is "No." Finding the gene, however, brings us another step closer to understanding just what goes wrong when this gene is inherited, and therefore how to strategize treatment or maybe even prevention.

Whether MJD will retain this name, or be called SCA3, remains to be resolved. A name is, after all, only a handle by which to identify something so that someone else may recognize it. The gene location and defect will be the ultimate differentiation for the ataxias no matter what they are called. The bottom line is ultimately what it will mean to the family members in terms of presymptomatic testing and treatment. Having identified a specific gene defect makes possible gene carrier and prenatal testing, as it is now possible to test a single individual for their gene carrier status. This, of course, makes relevant all of the issues of presymptomatic testing that were considered in the questionnaire that many of you completed for me back in 1991.

Testing for MJD/SCA3 is still in the research phase, however, which means no commercial laboratory is doing it as of this writing . A protocol for presymptomatic testing has been established for Huntington's disease (HD), another late onset neurological disease. This protocol addresses the inappropriateness of testing minors, as well as the necessity for testing to be accompanied by counseling to deal with the many practical and psychological issues. Once results from presymptomatic testing is given out, it is information that cannot be given back. Experience with HD suggests that at risk persons (that is, someone whose parent has or had the disease) who choose to learn their status rarely make major life changes, and that the majority of persons decline testing. This will likely change dramatically when a treatment becomes available.

Potential treatment is, of course, **the** main goal of genetic research. One kind of treatment, gene therapy, allows the substitution of a functional, working gene for a defective one. This approach is more likely to be useful in recessive disorders in which an affected individual has two nonworking genes - one inherited from each parent. Replacement of at least one of the genes can make up for the missing gene. With a dominant disease such as SCA, the disease is caused by only one gene of a pair being dysfunctional. It is, therefore, less likely that a replacement gene could restore function: one non-disease-causing gene already is present and is not compensating for the dysfunctional one.

An alternate approach to gene therapy would be to find a chemical that would compensate for whatever mistake is caused by the SCA gene. It may be possible, for instance, to prevent the accumulation of a harmful substance or to interfere with a biochemical pathway that leads to the death of a specific cell type. This strategy is being proposed for treatment of Amyotrophic Lateral Sclerosis (ALS) now that a causative gene has been identified.

In finding the gene, we have found the proverbial needle in the haystack! Our current technology can help us to understand the biological basis of this disease better than anyone has in the centuries since the disease first affected members of your family.
....And in understanding there is hope.

APPENDIX II

This is the kind of detail you might choose to delve into if you have an interest in the science. After I was diagnosed I wrote this for myself, as a way to organize how *alpha-synuclein* (SNCA) has revolutionized the field of Parkinson's research and, In Appendix III, promising approaches to new therapies.

Then it seemed to make sense to share it with others who are living with Parkinson's, and might want an understanding of what is meant when you hear a new approach to therapy discussed on Sixty Minutes or on the evening news.

Throughout Appendix II, I will use the simpler gene symbol, SNCA, in addition to *alpha-synuclein*.

Scientific Background
Contents

What Made The Contursi Kindred So Valuable

For the majority of Parkinson disease patients we do not find many living relatives with the disease. The Contursi kindred showed a clear-cut pattern of inheritance in which the disease passed from generation to generation, with each child of an affected individual at 50% risk of being affected. From the lessons of Gregor Mendel, the Father of Genetics, we know that when we see such a pattern of inheritance, a single dominant gene is causing the disorder. With such a family we need blood samples from at least ten affected persons, along with their unaffected relatives, in order to have enough mathematical power to locate a causative gene. In the Contursi family we had samples available from exactly ten affected persons!

How We Locate Genes

When DNA is passed on from parent to child, we know that it breaks and rearranges. This is the miracle of sexual reproduction, and is responsible for the infinite variation in traits between people. The closer two pieces of DNA are on a chromosome, the greater the chance that they will remain together during that process. When two such pieces of DNA remain unseparated as they are passed from one generation to the next, they are said to be *linked.*

Markers are random pieces of DNA that are found all throughout one's genetic material, or "genome." These markers have been found to have normal variations among perfectly healthy people, and as such have become tools in mapping human genes. Our 20–25,000 genes are divided up on 23 pairs of chromosomes. A given marker is always in the same place on everyone's chromosome so that, when looking for a disease-causing gene, a marker can serve as a known point on a chromosome. The faulty disease gene, whose location we are trying to determine, is then tested to see if it is consistently inherited along with a given marker.

Many markers have now been "mapped," meaning we know exactly where they are on which chromosome. Each chromosome has a central waist-like constriction with a long (q) arm and a short (p) arm. When stained and viewed under the microscope, each arm has a pattern of stripes that are numbered in a standardized way. A reference to a given marker, for instance on chromosome 2q1.4, lets another geneticist know exactly where to find it. When we infer the location of a disease gene from its having been inherited along with a given marker, the disease gene is said to be "localized," or mapped to a given chromosomal area.

Beginning in the 1980's short segments of DNA were cut into small pieces with chemical scissors and made radioactive to be used as markers for mapping genes. Then, by the mid 1990's, markers were identified that consisted of single units of DNA or "nucleotides" (Lander 1996). In 1996 Affymetrix revolutionized gene mapping with their GeneChips in which thousands of these single nucleotide polymorphism (SNP) markers could be analyzed on a single quartz chip less than 1" square. Once DNA is extracted from a person's blood cells, their entire complement of DNA can be put on a single chip for analysis. Gene chips have facilitated genome-wide association studies (GWAS) to look for susceptibility genes across the entire 23-chromosome-genome and across populations.

Before the gene chip, however, gel electrophoresis was laboriously used to identify SNPs. DNA samples from each person was loaded into one of many wells cut out on the top of a gel fixed in a large apparatus that held it vertically. The DNA filtered through the gel and separated by size in an electric current. Each person's DNA formed a column of different sized pieces, and the results were read from a photographic exposure of the gel (as seen in the photograph of Dr. Bill and Dr. Alice in Chapter 14). The DNA results were combined with the family relationships in a computer program designed for this purpose, and the likelihood that the marker and the disease were linked - inherited together because they are near each other on the same chromosome – was calculated.

A separate gel was run for each SNP, and, particularly in large families, multiple gels were needed to accommodate one well for each individual. Hundreds of markers were necessary to canvas the entire genome, so that localizing a single gene was extremely labor-intensive. On a good day our laboratory could run up to eight gels.

On a bad day, any number of errors in the process—a torn gel, for instance—could render one or more of the eight gels unusable.

How We Mapped the Contursi Kindred Gene

Mihaelis Polymeropoulos's laboratory had been working on a disease called Wolfram syndrome, which his laboratory had mapped to chromosome 4. Because many chromosome 4 markers used in the Wolfram experiments were already being used in his laboratory, they were the first markers to be run against the Contursi kindred samples. By a stroke of luck, some of these markers were consistently inherited along with the disease-causing gene, and the gene in the Contursi family was determined to be on the long arm of chromosome 4 (4q21-q23).

How We Identified the PARK1 Mutation

Once we know *where* a disease gene is, the next step is to identify *what it does.* We begin this by searching databases of genes to find ones that map to the same area. Sometimes initial gene localizations narrow the search to a region containing as many as 100 genes. Each of these genes needs to be considered to see if it could logically play a role in the disease pathology. Just as recipes contain the directions for the preparation of given dishes, genes hold the directions for the preparation of proteins. A gene for a protein that is found in the brain, then, is a good candidate for playing a role in a neurological disorder, while a gene for a protein found in the heart, is a good candidate for a cardiac disorder, and so forth.

The last, and sometimes most difficult, step is to actually *prove* a protein's involvement in the disease in question. To implicate a protein in a given disease, geneticists frequently extrapolate from the role of the equivalent gene product in another species. One protein, whose gene mapped to the area of chromosome 4q where the Contursi kindred gene mapped, was *alpha-synuclein* (SNCA) but in 1996 not much was known about it. In 1995, *synelfin,* the equivalent of SNCA in the zebra finch, had been reported to be involved in song learning (George, Jin et al. 1995). Rat synuclein had been shown to share 95% of its sequence with its human counterpart

(Campion, Martin et al. 1995). The fact that nature had conserved this protein between species suggested that it was an important brain protein, and therefore a good candidate for involvement in a neurological disorder.

SNCA had been purified from the senile plaques of Alzheimer's disease brains, but screening of patients with familial early-onset Alzheimer's had not revealed any mutations in the synuclein gene (Uéda, Fukushima et al. 1993). However, when Mihaelis's lab screened the Contursi DNA samples for mutations in the SNCA gene, an A53T mutation was consistently found in the individuals that were affected with PD, and it was absent in the unaffected persons.

Amino acids are strung together like beads to make up a protein. The A53T mutation found in the Contursi kindred changes the 53rd amino acid *from* Alanine *to* Threonine. As the first mutation to be reported for Parkinson disease, it was designated PARK1. We soon learned that the equivalent of the human mutation occurred naturally (referred to as the 'wild type') in both the finch and the rat, but neither animal had any characteristics that looked like human PD.

The location of a protein in the body can further strengthen the case for its disease involvement. The protein, SNCA, had been found to be associated with membrane structures in the brain regions that were prone to degeneration in Alzheimer's disease. We came to learn as well that the location of SNCA in the rat brain coincided with the areas of the brain that are affected in PD. This was an 'aha' moment in the convergence of Alzheimer's and Parkinson's for me and for my colleagues.

Immediately after our 1997 report of the A53T mutation for Parkinson's, SNCA was demonstrated to be the major component of Lewy bodies, the hallmark of human Parkinson's pathology (Spillantini, Schmidt et al. 1997). Mutations in proteins that break down SNCA were then reported in PD (Kitada, Asakawa et al. 1998, Leroy, Boyer et al. 1998), and the central role SNCA played in causing PD was further confirmed by reports of additional mutations in the SNCA gene in German and Spanish families (Kruger, Kuhn et al. 1998, Zarranz, Alegre et al. 2004).

The BIG Picture: How the Discovery of The PARK1 Mutation in Alpha-Synuclein (SNCA) Has Transformed PD Research

In the years since our discovery of the PARK1 mutation, a dramatic shift in understanding of Parkinson disease has taken place, from that of an environmentally mediated condition to a disease with a significant genetic component. The extremes of a genetic and apparently sporadic PD can be considered on a continuum, and this underlies the importance of genetic findings in understanding how sporadic disease develops (Devine and Lewis 2008).

It was another seven years before a mutation in the LRRK2 (leucine-rich repeat kinase 2) gene, also known as dardarin, was reported as PARK8 (Paisán-Ruíz, Jain et al. 2004). Humans have hundreds of "kinases," which are enzymes that add a phosphate group to another molecule and these are key to controlling complex cellular processes. Like SNCA mutations, LRRK2 mutations are inherited in a dominant manner and result in typical PD but, on autopsy, they can produce *either* Lewy bodies or "neurofibrillary tangles" (NFTs). NFTs are aggregates of a protein called *tau* that are found inside brain cells, and are a hallmark of Alzheimer disease brains. The occurance of Lewy bodies or NFTs with LRRK2 mutations suggests that SNCA and tau may both be downstream targets of LRRK2, linked to the dysregulation of their phosphorylation (Devine and Lewis 2008).

LRRK2 mutations turned out to be a common cause of PD, accounting for up to 10% of familial cases with dominant PD, and found in 10--30% of Ashkenazi Jews with PD. When Google co-founder, Sergey Brin discovered that he and his PD-affected mother both carried an LRRK2 mutation, he was able to bring to bear huge amounts of resources to promote the study of modifiers that affect the expression of the LRRK2 mutations and the development of therapeutics.

The Brin Wojcicki Foundation and The Michael J. Fox Foundation for Parkinson's Research have partnered in developing, and making public, a renewable source of monoclonal antibodies which are used to detect specific proteins, such as LRRK2, that are naturally present in small amounts. This arrangement avoids the issue of property rights that can unduly delay research progress, and will help to clarify the localization and distribution of LRRK2 in the brains.

In addition to PARK1 and PARK8, eleven Parkinson disease-causing genes have been identified, and a number of additional chromosomal locations have been mapped for which the genes remain to be identified. Other genes are associated with "susceptibility" to PD in which a gene is thought to contribute to causation. The chart below lists the genes identified as of this writing. Causation is listed as either autosomal dominant (AD), autosomal recessive (AR), unidentified, or as an association. These are continually updated on PD databases (http://www.pdgene.org and http://www.molgen.ua.ac.be/PDmutDB).

	Gene	location	caused by:
PARK1	SNCA	4q22.1	AD mutation
PARK2	PRKN	6q25.2-q27	AR mutation
PARK3	??	2p13	
PARK4	SNCA	4q22.1	triplication
PARK5	UCHL1	4p14	AD mutation
PARK6	PINK1	1p36	AR mutation
PARK7	DJ1	1p36	AR mutation
PARK8	LRRK2	12q12	AD mutation
PARK9	ATP13A2	1p36.13	AR mutation
PARK10	??	1p34-p32	
PARK11	GIGYF2	2q37	AD mutation
PARK12	??	Xq21-q25	
PARK13	HTRA2	2p12	AD mutation
PARK14	PLA2G6	22q13	AR mutation
PARK15	FBXO7	22q12-q13	AR mutation
PARK16	??	1q32	
PARK17	VPS35	16q11.2	AD mutation
PARK18	EIF4G1	3q27	AD mutation
	GBA	1q22	association
	MAPT	17q21.31	association
	MC1R	16q24.3	association
	ADH1C	4q23	association
	HLA-DRA	6p21.32	association
	GAK	4p16.3	association

PD Gene Mutations and Associations

Mitochondrial gene mutations have also been described. Mitochondria are tiny organelles within the cell that function as "energy factories." They have only 13 genes, whereas the nucleus within each cell has some 20–25,000 genes. Some of the nuclear genes in turn affect mitochondrial function, so that delineating their interaction becomes increasingly complicated. It will be interesting to see how the pathogenic pathways identified by elucidation of these individual mutations will enable us to move beyond our current, limited therapeutic repertoire, which is aimed at ameliorating the motor symptoms of PD.

Convergence of Theories of the Origin of Parkinson disease

As oxygen is the source of most of the brain's energy, brain cells, and dopamine producing cells in particular, consume a disproportionate amount of the body's oxygen. When cells utilize oxygen, mitochondria are depleted and oxygen radicals are generated. Oxidative stress refers to the toxic process within a cell as a result of the build up of these oxygen radicals. According to advocates of the mitochondrial theory, cell death in Parkinson's is caused when something interferes with its disposing of these toxic byproducts.

In the early 1980s, a severe and irreversible parkinsonian syndrome was diagnosed among young drug addicts in California. A nasty byproduct that formed during the preparation of their designer drugs caused a syndrome resembling the classic Parkinson's signs—tremor, slow movement, rigidity, and postural instability—that was relieved by antiparkinson's medications. The chemical is a brain poison, MPTP, that inhibits mitochondria, and the pattern of cell death that it causes closely resembles the pathology of Parkinson's. These "frozen addicts," as they came to be called, did not set out to contribute to research on Parkinson disease, but they ended up doing so in great measure. MPTP became a powerful tool in the creation of a mouse-model for the disease, a model that has contributed immeasurably to our understanding of PD.

Mitochondrial dysfunction in PD is supported by the known association of LRRK2 with the mitochondrial outer membrane (Devine and Lewis 2008). Further, several of the PD-causing genes

(PARK2, coding for Parkin, PARK6 for PINK1, and PARK7 for DJ-1)—are involved with mitochondrial function. The fact that they are inherited in an autosomal recessive manner—with a mutated gene passed down from each, unaffected, parent—suggests that some important cellular function is lost. By deciphering these diverse cellular pathways, one sees a number of ways to arrive at a similar disease entity—a meeting of geneticists and mitochodrialists.

Convergence of Neurodegenerative Disorders

We had known that protein aggregates occur in several late onset neurodegenerative disorders: extra-neuronal plaques and neurofibrillary tangles that are the hallmark of Alzheimer's; Lewy bodies which characterize Parkinson's; and the nuclear inclusions seen in Huntington's. It was subsequent to our describing the SNCA mutation in PD that researchers began to identify how these proteins aggregate, and that their respective diseases converge.

By 1997 one form of a neuronal protein, tau, had been found to be increased in Alzheimer disease (Conrad, Andreadis et al. 1997). With funding from the American Parkinson Disease Association, I was able to look at the presence of that tau form in samples from PD patients that we had in our lab and I found a similar increased frequency (Lazzarini, Golbe et al. 1997, Golbe, Lazzarini et al. 2001). Subsequent studies have supported the MAPT/tau locus on chromosome 17q21 as a major association for PD (Spencer, Plagnol et al. 2011).

SNCA and tau were later shown to interact to promote the folding of amyloid (Giasson, Forman et al. 2003) that forms the brain-clogging clumps indicative of Alzheimer's. Mutant Alzheimer and Parkinson's proteins have been shown to form indistinguishable fibrils (Lashuel, Hartley et al. 2002), and the beta-amyloid peptides characteristic of AD have been shown to promote aggregation of SNCA (Masliah, Rockenstein et al. 2001). For both tau and SNCA, it seems that the intermediate, oligomeric, form of the protein is most toxic, and that the final inclusions may represent the body's attempt to clear misfolded proteins.

In December of 2004, recognizing the commonalities among the disorders of protein aggregation, scientists gathered at the Cold Spring Harbor Laboratories for the third "Drug Discovery in Neurodegenerative Diseases" symposium. Their classification of neurodegenerative disorders according to their type of amyloid fibrils (synucleinopathies, amyloidopathies, or tauopathies) further lumped these diseases together.

Animal Models to Transgenics

The MPTP mouse model, created by introducing this toxic chemical byproduct into animal brains, shed light on PD that would have been impossible in humans, but the mice lack some Parkinson's-specific features. Further details of the disease pathology have been revealed by the deliberate construction of animals that have the specific genetic defects that are found in humans. Mice, flies, and even yeast that have been manipulated genetically are referred to as 'transgenic' animals because they can express gene products from different species.

Transgenic animals can be created: to make the mutated SNCA (called "knock-ins" because that specific gene is *added* to the animal); to have no SNCA at all (called "knock-outs"); or to express these in various combinations with other genes. Being able to alter the expression of specific gene products involved in a very complex sequence of events is providing a clearer picture of PD-specific pathways and accelerating discovery of promising therapeutic interventions.

Transgenic mice *deficient* in SNCA have been shown to be resistant to MPTP toxicity, so that MPTP toxicity is dependent on having SNCA. Conversely, *over expression* of SNCA in transgenic mice renders them more vulnerable to MPTP injury (Song, Shults et al. 2004), further strengthening the link between a genetic cause and mitochondrial dysfunction.

Transgenic mice that have the A53T mutation that we described, continue to inform our understanding of the mechanisms involved in SNCA toxicity (Oaks, Frankfurt et al. 2013). Various mutation combinations of LRRK2 crossbred with A53T transgenic mice showed that over-expression of LRRK2 alone did not cause neurodegeneration, but that it did accelerate SNCA aggregation. Conversely, knocking out LRRK2 delayed the progression of neuropathology in A53T mice. A synaptic vesicle protein, SNCA is transported by microtubule-based proteins to axonal terminals. In regulating this trafficking by stabilizing microtubule assembly, LRRK2 represents a potential therapeutic target (Lin, Parisiadou et al. 2009).

Transgenic mice with mutant SNCA show loss of dopamine cells just like in human Parkinson's. In one transgenic mouse line that was created to express both the A53T mutant SNCA and the heat-shock protein, HSP70, SNCA-caused cell loss was actually prevented (Auluck, Chan et al. 2002). SNCA is normally moved to a place where it is degraded and HSP70 is one of a class of "helper" molecules, known as a 'chaperone' that moves proteins within the cell. (Cuervo, Stefanis et al. 2004). The potential to prevent cell loss by turning on a single gene such as HSP70, becomes a promising avenue of further research—one that would not have been conceived without the understanding made possible by discovery of the initial SNCA mutation.

The ability to model abnormal SNCA accumulation enables us to study its consequences, clarify the molecular pathways involved, and identify potential therapeutic targets. Then, as novel therapeutic approaches are developed, these transgenic animal models provide an important tool to evaluating a drug's effect in slowing or stopping cell death.

APPENDIX III
Approaches to Treatment for Parkinson disease
Contents

Neurorestoration

Neuromodulation

Neurorestoration to Neuroprotection

    Modifiers of Protein Aggregation

    Antioxidants

    Inhibitors of Apoptosis (IAPs)

    Anti-inflammatory drugs

    Epigenetic Targets

Biomarkers

Drug Delivery Systems

    Gene Therapy

    Infusion

    The Trojan Horse Strategy

    Cell Replacement Therapies (CRTs)

Because cell death in Parkinson disease may be caused by SNCA aggregation, by dysfunction in the critical systems responsible for breakdown of proteins, or by reduced mitochondrial activity, each of these mechanisms presents us with a potential approach to therapeutic intervention. The cells of the *substantia nigra* seem to be especially vulnerable because dopamine metabolism produces highly reactive oxygen species (ROS) and results in increased oxidative stress (Obeso, Rodriguez-Oroz et al. 2010).

Neurorestoration

The first breakthrough in the treatment of Parkinson's came about forty years ago with the discovery that the drug, Sinemet, could replace the dopamine lost when dopamine-producing cells in the brain die. Sinemet is a combination of levodopa and carbidopa, and since going generic, is called carbidopa/levodopa. Levodopa, the precursor of dopamine, is used because dopamine itself cannot get through the "blood brain barrier," which functions to keep the brain environment stable; Carbidopa, prevents levodopa from being broken down before reaching the brain. While this drug seemed like the *magic bullet* that restored a PD patient's fluidity of movements, its effect diminishes after prolonged use. Eventually its use can be accompanied by excess involuntary flailing movements called *dyskinesias.* Treating Parkinson's then becomes a delicate dosage-dance to facilitate the medication's effect without causing *dyskinesias.* A cadre of dopamine agonists (*helpers* if you will)—drugs like pramipexole, ropinirole, and others—have been utilized to modulate symptoms and forestall the need for carbidopa/levodopa.

Drug-induced *dyskinesias* are thought to result from dopamine being delivered in a pulsatile manner. Several approaches to provide more continuous dosing have been proven useful, including a slow release formulation, infusion pumps to deliver steady medication doses, and medications that prevent the breakdown of the needed dopamine.

Neuromodulation

Deep brain stimulation of one of the two areas of the brain involved in PD (the subthalamic nucleus and the globus pallidus interna) is known as a neuromodulatory approach to treatment—aimed at modifying the *function* of specific areas of the brain affected by Parkinson's. These are current and successful treatments, albeit not without surgical risk.

Neurorestoration to Neuroprotection

Delineation of the various pathways associated with single-gene mutations, and the observation that the symptoms of Parkinson disease extend well beyond the motoric, has led Parkinson's experts to believe that a more widespread underlying neuropathology accounts for the progressive disability that becomes increasingly resistant to current medical therapy. They urged moving beyond a focus on dopamine deficiency, to investigate the pathogenesis of the degeneration, to identify the mechanisms involved in protein aggregation, and to develop drugs specifically designed to target the abnormal pathways. By deciphering the pathogenic cascades leading to Parkinson's, they hope to be able to develop the tools to recover brain integrity once the process has begun, that is *neurorestoration*. Taking it one step further, one might hope to prevent the disease process via *neuroprotection*.

Recovery of neuronal function has been achieved in a mouse model of Huntington disease, and dopamine cell loss can be prevented in the fly model of Parkinson's. Given such potential, the following are some of the approaches which have come out of our increased understanding of these pathological pathways, and which may show efficacy in slowing or stopping cell death in Parkinson's.

Modifiers of Protein Aggregation

In the laboratory of Jim Gusella at Massachusetts General Hospital, where the Huntington disease gene was identified back in 1993, over 1,000 compounds were screened for the ability to stop aggregation of the mutant Huntingtin protein in cell culture. Ten compounds were identified. Two of the ten, one of which was celastrol, were also capable of reversing abnormal cellular localization (Wang, Gines et al. 2005).

Celastrol is an anti-inflammatory and antioxidant compound and an active component in Chinese herbal medicine. The literature reveals consideration of the use of celastrol therapy in such diverse disorders as ALS, asthma, Crohn's disease, and in cancer, as it also blocks the formation of new blood vessels. In animal models of

193

Parkinson's, celastrol was shown to significantly stop the loss of dopaminergic neurons when delivered prior to the cells being stressed. Studies show that celastrol effects its protection by activating the heat shock protein (HSP) within dopaminergic neurons, which brings us full circle to the demonstration that turning on the HSP gene can prevent SNCA cell loss. Heat shock proteins belong to a class of 'chaperones' that help other proteins fold. Because folding is key in the diseases in which proteins aggregate, understanding the behavior of these chaperones is key to understanding how to intervene to prevent protein aggregation.

Intrabodies, or intracellular antibodies, delivered into the cell nucleus to selectively bind a specific protein (see The Trojan Horse Strategy below), also have the potential for altering the folding, interactions, modifications, or subcellular localization of their targets. These reagents have been developed as therapeutics against cancer and HIV, and have demonstrated prolonged survival in the fly and other models of Huntington disease. Given the important role of SNCA, and the pathological nature of its over expression in Parkinson's, inhibition of its aberrant effects using anti-SNCA intrabodies could prove a viable molecular therapeutic approach for the synucleinopathies.

Antioxidants

One source of oxidative stress in PD is the breakdown of dopamine by monoamine oxidase (MAO). MAO-B inhibitors such as the drug, Deprenyl (selegiline) have been in the PD treatment repertoire since being approved by the FDA in 1979. While they do help maintain dopamine levels and continue to provide some manner of symptomatic relief, a role in neuroprotection remains elusive. A more specific MAO-B inhibitor, the drug rasagiline, has shown what appears to be a preventive effect on the progression of PD disability, but this drug is known to work also by enhancing the expression of antiapoptotic and neurotrophic factors (see below).

The neurotransmitter, glutamate, is one of a group of several *excitotoxins*, which appear to selectively kill neurons. Glutamate is a major effector of oxidative stress through activation of several different receptors. Blockage (antagonism) of the glutamate AMPA receptor is an emerging treatment approach that has been shown in primate models of PD to have antiparkinsonian and antidyskinetic effects. The drug talampanel was an early drug in this category.

Coenzyme Q10 (ubiquinone) is a vitamin-like substance that is being examined in the treatment of a variety of disorders that are primarily related to suboptimal cellular energy metabolism and oxidative injury: Huntington disease, macular degeneration and cardiac disease, among others. It has been shown to be safe and well tolerated, and in a preliminary study of eighty-patients that was designed to determine effective doses, it appeared to slow the progressive deterioration of function in PD. However, a subsequent Phase III clinical trial was halted due to lack of efficacy. Other candidates for targeting mitochondrial dysfunction include agents such as creatine and modulating pathways that regulate antioxidants (Chaturvedi and Beal 2013)

Inhibitors of Apoptosis

Since the early 1970s, programmed (*apoptotic*) cell death has been distinguished from *necrotic* cell death resulting from injury. Referred to as the "cell suicide program," apoptosis is the more efficient way for cells to die because inflammation is avoided and the cell is rapidly removed. Apoptosis operates by default when a cell is deprived of appropriate survival signals from neurotrophic factors and cytokines. Areas of the nervous system are variably dependent on nerve growth factor (NGF), brain derived neurotrophic factor (BDNF), and glial cell line-derived neurotrophic factor (GDNF) to avoid apoptosis. The replacement, or stimulation in the nervous system, of factors such as BDNF and GDNF is another therapeutic strategy (see gene therapy below).

It is now recognized that most apoptosis proceeds through the mitochondrial pathway and that it can be triggered by a bewildering array of situations. JNK (c-Jun N-terminal kinase) is a molecule that activates a cascade of genes involved in the cell death-signaling pathway. This convergence of apoptosis and oxidative stress is seen in Alzheimer's in which beta-amyloid was shown to kill cells by turning on JNK, which in turn squelches the cell's antioxidant defenses.

The production of cyclooxygenase-2 (COX-2) has been shown to be increased in the brains of both Alzheimer's and Parkinson's patients via the JNK pathway, and thus may represent an important step in the molecular events leading to neurodegeneration. COX-2 inhibition prevents MPTP-induced neurodegeneration in mice, not by mitigating inflammation, as one expects from an anti-inflammatory drug, but by preventing the formation of an oxidant species. The safety of COX-2 inhibitors, however, has become a hot button for the pharmaceutical companies.

Caspases are a family of proteases that have been recognized as markers of apoptotic pathway activity, and reported as a promising avenue for treatment for both Huntington disease and stroke. Simultaneous manipulation of several genes in transgenic animals, however, has clarified the steps in the process of apoptosis and shown caspases are involved in the later phase.

JNK activation of the cell-death pathway has been shown to *precede* both COX-2 and caspase activation so that inhibition of the JNK pathway blocks the very early (upstream) events of the death-signaling pathway. The drug, CEP1347 inhibits key signals that trigger apoptotic neuronal death by interfering with the JNK pathway. In both cell lines and in the mouse model of PD, CEP1347 had been shown to lessen degeneration. The Parkinson's Study Group, a multi-institutional group that has conducted many clinical trials of potential PD medications, demonstrated the safety and tolerability of CEP1347 in a short-term study. While a larger study, the Parkinson Research Examination of CEP-1347 Trial (PRECEPT), was disappointing, drugs like CEP1347, or its successors, offer a treatment strategy and the potential for actual recovery of neuronal function.

Anti-inflammatory Drugs

I would be remiss not mentioning inflammation as another potential area for drug targeting. Extracellular SNCA oligomers activate microglia that act (through NF-k beta) to produce reactive oxygen species and proinflammatory mediators, creating a feedback-loop of inflammation in microglia and astrocytes, which in turn act directly on dopaminergic neurons of the substantia nigra. A recent pathway-based analysis has indicated that immune-related genetic susceptibility to PD is likely to be more widespread than previously appreciated (Holmans, Moskvina et al. 2013)

Nurr1, like other transcription factors that are active early in development, is also involved late-onset diseases via dysregulation. Nurr1 suppresses this inflammatory response and represents yet another approach to therapeutic intervention. Interestingly, dextromethorphan, the simple ingredient in many cough syrups, has been shown to reduce the degeneration of dopaminergic neurons in cell culture, apparently inhibiting the inflammatory response.

Epigenetic Targets

"Epigenetic" describes mechanisms that modify expression levels of genes without necessarily modifying the DNA sequence. By silencing, increasing or reducing the expression of a gene in a given tissue they can have similar effects to those of pathological mutations. Once referred to as "junk" DNA, the many non-coding, regulatory DNA sequences are increasingly being recognized for the importance they play in neurodegenerative pathology. The current William Dow Lovett Professor of Neurology at the Robert Wood Johnson Medical School, Maral Mouradian, has contributed to clarifying the importance of microRNAs involved in regulation of gene expression and the potential to harness their negative control of SNCA therapeutically (Mouradian 2012).

Biomarkers

While the PRECEPT study failed to prove efficacy for CEPH1837, it proved useful in identifying a potential biomarker. Researchers found that Uric acid levels were inversely correlated with clinical progression in PD, also pointing to drugs to elevate urate as a potential therapeutic approach.

This serendipitous finding has led to a redesigning of large studies to be consistent with NIH's Roadmap for Clinical Research, in which "systematically accrued longitudinal data can be made available for public access, retrieved for analyses, and in turn applied to inform about more efficient and relevant clinical outcomes, improved diagnostic precision, biomarkers applicable to the trait and state of PD, and promising therapeutic interventions" (Kolata Aug 13, 2010). The Parkinson's Disease Data and Organizing Center (www.pd-doc.org), supported by the National Institute of Neurological Disorders and Stroke (NINDS) and administered by the University of Rochester, functions to organize and facilitate both clinical research and translational research, that is, going from the laboratory to the patient.

Besides suggesting drug targets, biomarker signatures will be increasingly important for monitoring the efficacy of newly developed drugs aimed at neurorestoration. Then, as we progress toward neuroprotective therapies, biomarkers will be critical in identifying persons for whom prevention is appropriate.

The 2010 finding of a biomarker signature in Alzheimer disease resulted from a broad collaboration of researchers from academia and industry and has set a precedent for PD researchers that was not lost on the Michael J. Fox Foundation. The foundation now supports a five-year Parkinson's Progression Markers Initiative (PPMI), an international consortium of PD researchers to identify biomarkers of Parkinson disease progression.

Drug Delivery Systems
Gene Therapy

In gene therapy, a virus can be used to transport genes directly into cells, something at which viruses are naturally adept. When the part of a virus that causes infection is disabled, it can be specifically engineered to carry genes with the recipes for specific proteins. The challenge is to deliver such a *viral vector* where it is needed—a specific part of the brain in the case of a neurological disorder.

One such approach by Ceregene in San Diego has been to

198

package the gene for neurturin (CER-130), a growth factor that acts much like GDNF, into a gutted virus and infuse that virus under pressure into a PD patient's putamen. Initial results showed modest expression of the gene, and trials to also include delivery to the *substantia nigra* were undertaken (Vastag 2010). Unfortunately this approach failed to reach the endpoint of improved UPDRS scores in Phase 2b clinical trials, but one must take into account that the subjects chosen were moderately advanced patients who were uncontrolled by conventional medications.

Another approach to gene therapy is to utilize RNA interference (RNAi). RNA is the molecule that processes DNA into protein. In the late 1990s small interfering segments of RNA (siRNA) were found to be useful as tools in the laboratory as they could be made to interfere with the expression of a specific gene. A siRNA binds to its complementary strand of RNA and prevents it from processing a protein. It thus creates a state of reduced gene expression, referred to as a *knockdown*. When RNAi took off as a potential treatment for cancers, new biotech companies jumped on the bandwagon. RNAi can also shut down viral genes in HIV, and shut down a factor in the development of abnormal blood vessels in eyes with age related macular degeneration.

For neurodegenerative disorders, small interfering RNA's (siRNAs) can be designed to specifically bind and turn down the formation of proteins such as SNCA that accumulate in a diseased brain. RNAi was originally thought to knockdown expression of a single specific gene, but recent data has shown it has some "cross-reaction" with other gene targets. While siRNA has been successful in a mouse model of Huntington's, the cross-reaction issues will also have to be clarified before RNAi could be considered as a viable therapeutic agent. Other challenges, such as developing effective delivery to the correct target cells, and finding a viral vector that works in non-dividing cells, remain when applying siRNA to the nervous system.

Infusion

Direct infusion of neurotrophic factors such as GDNF into the brain has been fraught with well-publicized safety issues. *Sixty Minutes* covered a Phase II clinical trial run by Amgen that was stopped suddenly. The drug was withdrawn from the forty-eight patients who had had pumps surgically implanted to deliver the medication directly into their brains, and the participating doctors were ordered to remove the pumps. Amgen claimed some monkeys showed brain lesions at high doses.

One of their doctor's told the spouse of a PD participant, "Well, you wouldn't want your husband to be brain damaged, right, from this drug?" to which the woman retorted, "My husband is already brain damaged." Despite the patients' promising to wave any rights to sue, and attempts by the courts to force Amgen to continue the GDNF treatment, the company did not relent. Amgen's consulting bioethicist admitted that recent lawsuits involving the safety of drugs like Vioxx were a factor in Amgen's decision-making process. We are left then with desperate patients—like my friend who paid out of pocket for a fetal transplant—caught in the middle.

Experiments varying the delivery system, including the development of a catheter, with which to deliver GDNF under pressure, led to the finding that neuronal fibers had in fact sprouted in a patient who had had functional improvement. Still, the problem of consistent delivery remains, as does the danger of collateral effects of GDNF in other areas of the brain.

The Trojan Horse Strategy

The potential of viral vectors to deliver intrabodies into the cell nucleus to selectively bind a specific protein prompted researchers to address the problem of getting across the blood brain barrier without the need for invasive surgery.

In a literal interpretation of the concept of 'designer-drug,' a group at Stanford came up with a unique strategy to block aggregation in Alzheimer's. Small beta-amyloid-inhibitor molecules cannot interfere with large protein surfaces, so the researchers created a beta-amyloid inhibiting drug tethered to a molecule that binds a chaperone. In a cell culture system this approach reduced beta-amyloid toxicity. The shear bulk of the larger chaperone/drug/beta-amyloid complex, they predicted, could prevent protein aggregation if only it could get into the brain (Gestwicki, Crabtree et al. 2004).

Launched in 2004, ArmaGen Technologies developed a small antibody against beta-amyloid that was fused to a monoclonal antibody against the human insulin receptor which served to ferry it across the blood brain barrier (Boado, Lu et al. 2010). In the capillaries that feed the brain, insulin receptors grab molecules of insulin and pull them into brain tissue. Thus these receptors make ideal transporters, pulling the antibody into the brain along with the insulin.

Returning to the promise of growth factors, ArmaGen developed a hybrid protein, AGT-190, which fuses the GDNF gene with an antibody. Injected into animal veins, the amount which arrives in the brain is commensurate with other small-molecule-brain-drugs which cross the blood brain barrier unassisted (Vastag 2010). The safety and specificity of this Trojan horse approach remains to be demonstrated.

Cell Replacement Therapies (CRTs)

As PD is primarily characterized by loss of midbrain substantia nigra dopaminergic (DA) neurons that project into the striatum, grafting DA-producing cells into the striatum is another approach to providing an ongoing source of the missing dopamine.

In the late 1990s, fetal cell transplants were touted as the way to replace the neurons that were dying. As fetal cell grafting required 6 to 7 ventral midbrains from 6 to 9 week old aborted human embryos to treat a single PD patient, the procedure generated considerable ethical controversy.

Further, fetal transplants in general have not lived up to the promise of earlier studies. Despite solid evidence for survival and function of the transplanted cells, the finding of Lewy bodies and *alpha-synuclein* aggregates within the grafted cells at autopsy suggested spread from the host tissue to the grafts. This unique mechanism of pathological progression has been likened to that for *prion* disorders in which a protein self-aggregates and transmits to unaffected cells (Olanow and Prusiner 2009). Such "permissive templating" would also have to be overcome before stem cell therapy could be viable.

While the approaches to therapeutic intervention discussed herein are by no means exhaustive, they exemplify the myriad of ways that the research into cellular pathways of known gene mutations has clarified our understanding of PD pathogenesis.

Back in 2004, when a diagnosis of PD radically altered my journey, *alpha-synuclein*-based therapeutics were but a hope:

> *The next generation of PD treatments will no doubt be based on research that would not have been possible without the identification of that first rare mutation in alpha-synuclein.*
>
> *(Pankratz and Foroud 2004)*

Now, as I conclude this writing, *alpha-synuclein* targeted Parkinson's drug development is a major focus of The Michael J. Fox Foundation and of the entire PD research community. According to the MJFF website, they have invested more than $47,000,000 in *alpha-synuclein*-targeted research to date.

The foundation has awarded funding to AFFiRiS AG, an Austria-based biotech company for the development of a vaccine targeting *alpha-synuclein* (Schneeberger, Mandler et al. 2012); to Dr. Braithwaite at Signum Biosciences to explore PP2A as a therapeutic target to decrease the phosphorylation of *alpha-synuclein* (Braithwaite, Voronkov et al. 2012); and to reMYND, a Belgian company that pioneered a new drug-discovery process, for the advancement of a novel drug candidate directed against *alpha-synuclein*-triggered-toxicity.

Further, they have funded a consortium to develop an imaging agent for *alpha*-synuclein that could serve as a biomarker in living PD brains, enabling diagnosis and monitoring of therapeutic response (Bagchi, Yu et al. 2013).

NOTES

Chapter 3: Diagnosis
1. (Golbe, Lazzarini, et al. 2001)

Chapter 8: Becoming a Professional
1. Because many of the lay organizations were established before the possessive form for diseases was officially eliminated in the 1980's, it remains possessive in the organization's official titles.

2. Rutgers Medical School was founded in 1966. In 1975, it became part of The University of Medicine and Dentistry of New Jersey, and was renamed, UMDNJ - In 2013 it changed again to become Rutgers Robert Wood Johnson Medical School.

Chapter 13: Ataxia is Not a Foreign Cab
1. Neurologists had long separated different *ataxias* based only on what they could see on clinical examination. But by the 1990s new genetic technology was allowing us to examine DNA samples from families in which there were many affected individuals, and to separate the *ataxias* based on the genes that cause them. They were then named sequentially: SCA1, SCA2, SCA3, SCA4 and counting.

2 (Lazzarini, Zimmerman Jr et al. 1992)

Chapter 15: The Boss and Parkinson Disease
1 (Golbe, Di Iorio et al. 1990)

2. (Lazzarini, Myers et al. 1994)

Chapter 16: Contursi
1. In a pedigree, males are indicated by squares and females, circles. Each person has a Roman numeral to indicate the generation of which she/he is a part, plus an Arabic number to indicate his or her unique position within that generation.

2. (Polymeropoulos, Higgins et al. 1996)

Chapter 17: Discovery of PARK1
1. (Polymeropoulos, Lavedan et al. 1997)

2. (Spillantini, Schmidt et al. 1997).

Postscript: Gone to the Birds
1. (Warren, Clayton et al. 2010).

2. (Simonyan, Horwitz et al. 2012).

3. (Hilliard, Miller et al. 2012)

4. (Kurz, Wohr et al. 2010).

5. (Agate, Scott et al. 2009).

Epilogue: *Alpha*-synuclein and Me
1. 1-methyl-4-phenyl-1,2,3,6-tetrahydropyridine

2. (Nicklas, Vyas et al. 1985).

3. (Golbe, Di Iorio et al. 1990),

4. (Pankratz, Beecham et al. 2012).

5. (Freeman, Cedillos et al. 2013).

REFERENCES

(June 24, 2010). "Emerging Therapies: From Microscope to Marketplace, Parkinson's Action Network (PAN) ".

Agate, R. J., B. B. Scott, B. Haripal, C. Lois and F. Nottebohm (2009). "Transgenic songbirds offer an opportunity to develop a genetic model for vocal learning." Proc Natl Acad Sci U S A **106**(42): 17963-17967.

Auluck, P. K., H. Y. E. Chan, J. Q. Trojanowski, V. M.-Y. Lee and N. M. Bonini (2002). "Chaperone Suppression of α-Synuclein Toxicity in a Drosophila Model for Parkinson's Disease." Science **295**(5556): 865-868.

Bagchi, D. P., L. Yu, J. S. Perlmutter, J. Xu, R. H. Mach, Z. Tu and P. T. Kotzbauer (2013). "Binding of the radioligand SIL23 to alpha-synuclein fibrils in Parkinson disease brain tissue establishes feasibility and screening approaches for developing a Parkinson disease imaging agent." PLoS One **8**(2): e55031.

Boado, R. J., J. Z. Lu, E. K.-W. Hui and W. M. Pardridge (2010). "IgG-single chain Fv fusion protein therapeutic for alzheimer's disease: Expression in CHO cells and pharmacokinetics and brain delivery in the rhesus monkey." Biotechnology and Bioengineering **105**(3): 627-635.

Braithwaite, S. P., M. Voronkov, J. B. Stock and M. M. Mouradian (2012). "Targeting phosphatases as the next generation of disease modifying therapeutics for Parkinson's disease." Neurochem Int **61**(6): 899-906.

Campion, D., C. Martin, R. Heilig, F. Charbonnier, V. Moreau, J. M. Flaman, J. L. Petit, D. Hannequin, A. Brice and T. Frebourg† (1995). "The NACP/synuclein gene: chromosomal assignment and screening for alterations in Alzheimer disease." Genomics **26**(2): 254-257.

Chaturvedi, R. K. and M. F. Beal (2013). "Mitochondria targeted therapeutic approaches in Parkinson's and Huntington's diseases." Mol Cell Neurosci **55**: 101-114.

Conrad, C., A. Andreadis, J. Q. Trojanowski, D. W. Dickson, D. Kang, X. Chen, W. Wiederholt, L. Hansen, E. Masliah, L. J. Thal, R. Katzman, Y. Xia and T. Saitoh (1997). "Genetic evidence for the involvement of tau in progressive supranuclear palsy." Ann Neurol **41**(2): 277-281.

Cuervo, A. M., L. Stefanis, R. Fredenburg, P. T. Lansbury and D. Sulzer (2004). "Impaired Degradation of Mutant α-Synuclein by Chaperone-Mediated Autophagy." Science **305**(5688): 1292-1295.

Devine, M. J. and P. A. Lewis (2008). "Emerging pathways in genetic Parkinson's disease: tangles, Lewy bodies and LRRK2." FEBS Journal **275**(23): 5748-5757.

Freeman, D., R. Cedillos, S. Choyke, Z. Lukic, K. McGuire, S. Marvin, A. M. Burrage, S. Sudholt, A. Rana, C. O'Connor, C. M. Wiethoff and E. M. Campbell (2013). "Alpha-synuclein induces lysosomal rupture and cathepsin dependent reactive oxygen species following endocytosis." PLoS One **8**(4): e62143.

George, J. M., H. Jin, W. S. Woods and D. F. Clayton (1995). "Characterization of a novel protein regulated during the critical period for song learning in the zebra finch." Neuron **15**(2): 361-372.

Gestwicki, J. E., G. R. Crabtree and I. A. Graef (2004). "Harnessing Chaperones to Generate Small-Molecule Inhibitors of Amyloid ß Aggregation." Science **306**(5697): 865-869.

Giasson, B. I., M. S. Forman, M. Higuchi, L. I. Golbe, C. L. Graves, P. T. Kotzbauer, J. Q. Trojanowski and V. M.-Y. Lee (2003). "Initiation and Synergistic Fibrillization of Tau and Alpha-Synuclein." Science **300**(5619): 636-640.

Golbe, L. I., G. Di Iorio, V. Bonavita, D. C. Miller and R. C. Duvoisin (1990). "A large kindred with autosomal dominant Parkinson's disease." Ann Neurol **27**(3): 276-282.

Golbe, L. I., A. M. Lazzarini, J. R. Spychala, W. G. Johnson, E. S. Stenroos, M. H. Mark and J. I. Sage (2001). "The tau A0 allele in Parkinson's disease." Movement Disorders **16**(3): 442-447.

Hilliard, A. T., J. E. Miller, S. Horvath and S. A. White (2012). "Distinct neurogenomic states in basal ganglia subregions relate differently to singing behavior in songbirds." PLoS Comput Biol **8**(11): e1002773.

Holmans, P., V. Moskvina, L. Jones, M. Sharma, A. Vedernikov, F. Buchel, M. Sadd, J. M. Bras, F. Bettella, N. Nicolaou, J. Simon-Sanchez, F. Mittag, J. R. Gibbs, C. Schulte, A. Durr, R. Guerreiro, D. Hernandez, A. Brice, H. Stefansson, K. Majamaa, T. Gasser, P. Heutink, N. W. Wood, M. Martinez, A. B. Singleton, M. A. Nalls, J.

Hardy, H. R. Morris and N. M. Williams (2013). "A pathway-based analysis provides additional support for an immune-related genetic susceptibility to Parkinson's disease." Hum Mol Genet **22**(5): 1039-1049.

Kitada, T., S. Asakawa, N. Hattori, H. Matsumine, Y. Yamamura, S. Minoshima, M. Yokochi, Y. Mizuno and N. Shimizu (1998). "Mutations in the parkin gene cause autosomal recessive juvenile parkinsonism." Nature **392**(6676): 605-608.

Kruger, R., W. Kuhn, T. Muller, D. Woitalla, M. Graeber, S. Kosel, H. Przuntek, J. T. Epplen, L. Schols and O. Riess (1998). "Ala30Pro mutation in the gene encoding alpha-synuclein in Parkinson's disease." Nat Genet **18**(2): 106-108.

Kurz, A., M. Wohr, M. Walter, M. Bonin, G. Auburger, S. Gispert and R. K. Schwarting (2010). "Alpha-synuclein deficiency affects brain Foxp1 expression and ultrasonic vocalization." Neuroscience **166**(3): 785-795.

Lander, E. S. (1996). "The new genomics: global views of biology." Science **274**(5287): 536-539.

Lashuel, H. A., D. Hartley, B. M. Petre, T. Walz and P. T. Lansbury (2002). "Neurodegenerative disease: Amyloid pores from pathogenic mutations." Nature **418**(6895): 291-291.

Lazzarini, A., T. R. Zimmerman Jr, W. G. Johnson and R. C. Duvoisin (1992). "A 17th-century founder gives rise to a large North American pedigree of autosomal dominant spinocerebellar ataxia not linked to the SCA1 locus on chromosome 6." Neurology **42**(11): 2118-2124.

Lazzarini, A. M., L. Golbe, D. Dickson, R. Duvoisin and W. Johnson (1997). "Tau intronic polymorphism in Parkinson's Disease and Progressive Supranuclear Palsy." Neurology **48**: A427.

Lazzarini, A. M. M., R. H. P. Myers, T. R. J. M. D. Zimmerman, M. H. M. Mark, L. I. M. Golbe, J. I. M. Sage, W. G. M. Johnson and R. C. M. Duvoisin (1994). "A clinical genetic study of Parkinson's disease: Evidence for dominant transmission." Neurology **44**(3, Part 1): 499-506.

Leroy, E., R. Boyer, G. Auburger, B. Leube, G. Ulm, E. Mezey, G. Harta, M. J. Brownstein, S. Jonnalagada, T. Chernova, A. Dehejia, C. Lavedan, T. Gasser, P. J. Steinbach, K. D. Wilkinson and M. H.

Polymeropoulos (1998). "The ubiquitin pathway in Parkinson's disease." Nature **395**(6701): 451-452.

Lin, X., L. Parisiadou, X.-L. Gu, L. Wang, H. Shim, L. Sun, C. Xie, C.-X. Long, W.-J. Yang, J. Ding, Z. Z. Chen, P. E. Gallant, J.-H. Tao-Cheng, G. Rudow, J. C. Troncoso, Z. Liu, Z. Li and H. Cai (2009). "Leucine-Rich Repeat Kinase 2 Regulates the Progression of Neuropathology Induced by Parkinson's-Disease-Related Mutant α-synuclein." Neuron **64**(6): 807-827.

Masliah, E., E. Rockenstein, I. Veinbergs, Y. Sagara, M. Mallory, M. Hashimoto and L. Mucke (2001). "β-Amyloid peptides enhance α-synuclein accumulation and neuronal deficits in a transgenic mouse model linking Alzheimer's disease and Parkinson's disease." Proceedings of the National Academy of Sciences **98**(21): 12245-12250.

Mouradian, M. M. (2012). "MicroRNAs in Parkinson's disease." Neurobiol Dis **46**(2): 279-284.

Nicklas, W. J., I. Vyas and R. E. Heikkila (1985). "Inhibition of NADH-linked oxidation in brain mitochondria by 1-methyl-4-phenyl-pyridine, a metabolite of the neurotoxin, 1-methyl-4-phenyl-1,2,5,6-tetrahydropyridine." Life Sci **36**(26): 2503-2508.

Oaks, A. W., M. Frankfurt, D. I. Finkelstein and A. Sidhu (2013). "Age-dependent effects of A53T alpha-synuclein on behavior and dopaminergic function." PLoS One **8**(4): e60378.

Obeso, J. A., M. C. Rodriguez-Oroz, C. G. Goetz, C. Marin, J. H. Kordower, M. Rodriguez, E. C. Hirsch, M. Farrer, A. H. Schapira and G. Halliday (2010). "Missing pieces in the Parkinson's disease puzzle." Nat Med **16**(6): 653-661.

Olanow, C. W. and S. B. Prusiner (2009). "Is Parkinson's disease a prion disorder?" Proc Natl Acad Sci U S A **106**(31): 12571-12572.

Paisán-Ruíz, C., S. Jain, E. W. Evans, W. P. Gilks, J. Simón, M. van der Brug, A. L. de Munain, S. Aparicio, A. M. n. Gil, N. Khan, J. Johnson, J. R. Martinez, D. Nicholl, I. M. Carrera, A. S. Peňa, R. de Silva, A. Lees, J. F. Martí-Massó, J. Pérez-Tur, N. W. Wood and A. B. Singleton (2004). "Cloning of the Gene Containing Mutations that Cause PARK8-Linked Parkinson's Disease." Neuron **44**(4): 595-600.

Pankratz, N., G. W. Beecham, A. L. DeStefano, T. M. Dawson, K. F.

Doheny, S. A. Factor, T. H. Hamza, A. Y. Hung, B. T. Hyman, A. J. Ivinson, D. Krainc, J. C. Latourelle, L. N. Clark, K. Marder, E. R. Martin, R. Mayeux, O. A. Ross, C. R. Scherzer, D. K. Simon, C. Tanner, J. M. Vance, Z. K. Wszolek, C. P. Zabetian, R. H. Myers, H. Payami, W. K. Scott and T. Foroud (2012). "Meta-analysis of Parkinson's disease: identification of a novel locus, RIT2." Ann Neurol 71(3): 370-384.

Pankratz, N. and T. Foroud (2004). "Genetics of Parkinson disease." NeuroRx 1(2): 235-242.

Polymeropoulos, M. H., J. J. Higgins, L. I. Golbe, W. G. Johnson, S. E. Ide, G. D. Iorio, G. Sanges, E. S. Stenroos, L. T. Pho, A. A. Schaffer, A. M. Lazzarini, R. L. Nussbaum and R. C. Duvoisin (1996). "Mapping of a Gene for Parkinson's Disease to Chromosome 4q21-q23." Science 274(5290): 1197-1199.

Polymeropoulos, M. H., C. Lavedan, E. Leroy, S. E. Ide, A. Dehejia, A. Dutra, B. Pike, H. Root, J. Rubenstein, R. Boyer, E. S. Stenroos, S. Chandrasekharappa, A. Athanassiadou, T. Papapetropoulos, W. G. Johnson, A. M. Lazzarini, R. C. Duvoisin, G. Di Iorio, L. I. Golbe and R. L. Nussbaum (1997). "Mutation in the α-Synuclein Gene Identified in Families with Parkinson's Disease." Science 276(5321): 2045-2047.

Schneeberger, A., M. Mandler, F. Mattner and W. Schmidt (2012). "Vaccination for Parkinson's disease." Parkinsonism Relat Disord 18 Suppl 1: S11-13.

Simonyan, K., B. Horwitz and E. D. Jarvis (2012). "Dopamine regulation of human speech and bird song: a critical review." Brain Lang 122(3): 142-150.

Song, D. D., C. W. Shults, A. Sisk, E. Rockenstein and E. Masliah (2004). "Enhanced substantia nigra mitochondrial pathology in human α-synuclein transgenic mice after treatment with MPTP." Experimental Neurology 186(2): 158-172.

Spencer, C. C., V. Plagnol, A. Strange, M. Gardner, C. Paisan-Ruiz, G. Band, R. A. Barker, C. Bellenguez, K. Bhatia, H. Blackburn, J. M. Blackwell, E. Bramon, M. A. Brown, M. A. Brown, D. Burn, J. P. Casas, P. F. Chinnery, C. E. Clarke, A. Corvin, N. Craddock, P. Deloukas, S. Edkins, J. Evans, C. Freeman, E. Gray, J. Hardy, G. Hudson, S. Hunt, J. Jankowski, C. Langford, A. J. Lees, H. S. Markus, C. G. Mathew, M. I. McCarthy, K. E. Morrison, C. N. Palmer, J. P. Pearson, L. Peltonen, M.

Pirinen, R. Plomin, S. Potter, A. Rautanen, S. J. Sawcer, Z. Su, R. C. Trembath, A. C. Viswanathan, N. W. Williams, H. R. Morris, P. Donnelly and N. W. Wood (2011). "Dissection of the genetics of Parkinson's disease identifies an additional association 5' of SNCA and multiple associated haplotypes at 17q21." Hum Mol Genet 20(2): 345-353.

Spillantini, M. G., M. L. Schmidt, V. M. Y. Lee, J. Q. Trojanowski, R. Jakes and M. Goedert (1997). "[alpha]-Synuclein in Lewy bodies." Nature 388(6645): 839-840.

Uéda, K., H. Fukushima, E. Masliah, Y. Xia, A. Iwai, M. Yoshimoto, D. A. Otero, J. Kondo, Y. Ihara and T. Saitoh (1993). "Molecular cloning of cDNA encoding an unrecognized component of amyloid in Alzheimer disease." Proceedings of the National Academy of Sciences 90(23): 11282-11286.

Vastag, B. (2010). "Biotechnology: Crossing the barrier." Nature 466(7309): 916-918.

Wang, J., S. Gines, M. E. MacDonald and J. F. Gusella (2005). "Reversal of a full-length mutant huntingtin neuronal cell phenotype by chemical inhibitors of polyglutamine-mediated aggregation." BMC Neurosci 6: 1.

Warren, W. C., D. F. Clayton, H. Ellegren, A. P. Arnold, L. W. Hillier, A. Kunstner, S. Searle, S. White, A. J. Vilella, S. Fairley, A. Heger, L. Kong, C. P. Ponting, E. D. Jarvis, C. V. Mello, P. Minx, P. Lovell, T. A. Velho, M. Ferris, C. N. Balakrishnan, S. Sinha, C. Blatti, S. E. London, Y. Li, Y. C. Lin, J. George, J. Sweedler, B. Southey, P. Gunaratne, M. Watson, K. Nam, N. Backstrom, L. Smeds, B. Nabholz, Y. Itoh, O. Whitney, A. R. Pfenning, J. Howard, M. Volker, B. M. Skinner, D. K. Griffin, L. Ye, W. M. McLaren, P. Flicek, V. Quesada, G. Velasco, C. Lopez-Otin, X. S. Puente, T. Olender, D. Lancet, A. F. Smit, R. Hubley, M. K. Konkel, J. A. Walker, M. A. Batzer, W. Gu, D. D. Pollock, L. Chen, Z. Cheng, E. E. Eichler, J. Stapley, J. Slate, R. Ekblom, T. Birkhead, T. Burke, D. Burt, C. Scharff, I. Adam, H. Richard, M. Sultan, A. Soldatov, H. Lehrach, S. V. Edwards, S. P. Yang, X. Li, T. Graves, L. Fulton, J. Nelson, A. Chinwalla, S. Hou, E. R. Mardis and R. K. Wilson (2010). "The genome of a songbird." Nature 464(7289): 757-762.

Zarranz, J. J., J. Alegre, J. C. Gómez-Esteban, E. Lezcano, R. Ros, I.

Ampuero, L. Vidal, J. Hoenicka, O. Rodriguez, B. Atarés, V. Llorens, E. G. Tortosa, T. del Ser, D. G. Muñoz and J. G. de Yebenes (2004). "The new mutation, E46K, of α-synuclein causes parkinson and Lewy body dementia." <u>Annals of Neurology</u> 55(2): 164-173.

ABOUT THE AUTHOR

While raising a son and daughter, now adult professionals, Alice Lazzarini earned an MS in Genetic Counseling at Rutgers University, followed, at the age of fifty-five, by a PhD in Cell and Developmental Biology. She has had a long career practicing genetic counseling, coordinating a statewide program for Huntington disease families [the New Jersey's Huntington Disease Family Service Center], doing research in neurogenetic disorders, as well as in developing clinical trials for Parkinson disease drugs.

Named one of the 20 top authors in Parkinson disease research (1996-2006), she is known as well for research in the genetics of Huntington disease, restless legs syndrome, and ataxia, and has contributed over 75 papers and abstracts to the scientific literature.

In 1994 she published a paper on the genetics of Parkinson's disease that helped to turn the tide of thinking within the neurology community toward accepting a genetic component to the cause of Parkinson's disease. In 1996 she was part of an international team that reported the location on chromosome four of the first Parkinson's disease-causing gene mutation in a large family from Contursi, Italy. In 1997, her team identified the Contursi family's mutation (named "PARK1") in the *alpha-synuclein* gene (SNCA). Shorty thereafter Dr. Lazzarini was first to report the association of Parkinson's with the protein *tau*.

The discovery that SNCA builds up in the brains of everyone with PD has led to the first drug trial to leverage these genetic breakthroughs. On July 31' 2014, the Austrian biotech company, AFFiRiS AG, announced the results of a trial to test a drug designed to counter SNCA's detrimental effect in the brains of people with Parkinson's. A small, primarily safety study, its success allows this new treatment approach to move onto larger studies.

Finding herself diagnosed with the very disease for which she helped find a causative gene, she now experiences the race toward the development of new treatments with an additional sense of urgency.

CPSIA information can be obtained at www.ICGtesting.com
Printed in the USA
LVOW08s1719230115

424091LV00011B/215/P